The Social Psychology of
Communication Impairment

The Social Psychology of Communication Impairment

SHELAGH BRUMFITT PhD, M.PHIL, Reg MRCSLT

Department of Human Communication Sciences
University of Sheffield

WHURR PUBLISHERS
LONDON

© 1999 Whurr Publishers Ltd
First published 1999 by
Whurr Publishers Ltd
19b Compton Terrrace
London N1 2UN England, and 325 Chestnut Street,
Philadelphia PA 19106, USA

British Library Cataloguing in Publication Data
A catalogue record for this book is available from the
British Library.

ISBN 1 86156 095 8

Printed and bound in Great Britain by Athenaeum Press Ltd,
Gateshead, Tyne & Wear.

Contents

Preface

It is something of a mystery that the study of communication impairment has failed to include the influence of both social and health psychology in its core understanding. The discipline of neuropsychology has given remarkable insights into language impairments, yet we have little knowledge about what influences the behaviour of *people* with language impairments. What does it feel like to be a child with a language problem? What makes the child feel better? What makes the child feel worse?

Therapeutic approaches are expected to demonstrate change in the individual. However we need to be clearer about which factors affect the capacity for change in the communicatively impaired person. Interestingly, few texts on social psychology or health psychology refer to the predicaments of people with communication problems. Yet many other groups of people are used in psychological studies, such as people with Aids, diabetes, kidney disease and heart conditions. Somehow, communicatively impaired people have been overlooked. This may be because interviewing and questioning people with communication problems is very difficult. Well-used measures for other groups of people may be inappropriate and no one has modified these to make them appropriate.

This book is intended to redress the balance, in order to recognise the importance of social behaviour in the complexity of the communication problem. The following chapters are intended to explore the aspects of social and health psychology which are relevant to the communicatively impaired speaker and look at ways in which we can understand their predicament more fully.

Ackowledgements

I would like to thank all my colleagues in the Department of Human Communication Sciences at the University of Sheffield for helpful advice about reading sources.

The stages of development given on pages 44–45 are from Identity and the Life Cycle by Erik H Erikson. Copyright © 1980 by W.W. Norton & Company, Inc. Copyright © 1959 by International Universities Press, Inc. and are reprinted by permission of W.W. Norton & Company, Inc.

Introduction: Social Psychology and Health Psychology

Psychology covers many areas of interest from neuropsychology to the study of the unconscious. Social and health psychology are both directed at the core aspects of psychological understanding; that is, the behaviour of human beings. Social psychology looks at the individual in the social context and health psychology looks at a more specific aspect of how human beings behave in health care situations and what factors may affect the individual's response to health care.

Both areas have long and respected histories in the psychological literature. This makes sense. Of course we want to know why people are different from each other and how they might be the same. What is the most and least effective way to influence a person's behaviour? What makes one person more likely to take advice than another? How does group behaviour differ from individual behaviour? How do we understand ourselves?

Tesser (1995) discusses the history of social psychology and notes that the first social psychological experiment is usually attributed to Triplett (1898). In this experiment he had children wind fishing reels as fast as they could. Triplett found that the children who were in the company of other children would wind their reels faster than if they were alone. The significance of this experiment is that it determined the importance of looking at what influences behaviour. Clearly an understanding of behavioural influences would have implications for all of society. Although not all of this understanding may be put to good use (selling items to people who are known to be more vulnerable than others is clearly not good practice), there is no doubt that social good can come from understanding why people behave in certain ways.

Chapter 1
Self and Identity

Overview

From this chapter you will be able to:

- define the concept of the self
- understand the relationship between self-knowledge and other related features such as memory, behaviour and development
- develop insight into the way theories about self and identity can be applied in a speech and language therapy context.

Introduction

Although we may not be consciously aware of it, we all use definitions to describe ourselves. You work in a university, say. You may go in one day to sort out some reading and somehow just not manage to get anything organised. The library is busy, you are feeling tired, the subject is not too interesting. At the end of the day you go home and feel despondent about having achieved so little. When you reflect on what happened you might come to the conclusion that you just do not feel 'like yourself' today. In our everyday culture this is a frequently used saying: 'I'm just not feeling myself today'. We all recognise it and have probably used it on numerous occasions.

What is implied in this saying is that you recognise that you have a 'known' self. When you deviate from this you can, to a certain extent, recognise this too. Thus, you know yourself and you know that you are not someone else. You have a conscious awareness that you are separate. It would seem that the notion of having a self or identity is embedded in all our consciousnesses, even though we might not make this explicit to ourselves or other people.

Children are brought up hearing descriptions about themselves all the time. They are told if they are 'good' or 'naughty'. These labels may be used to develop a sense of self-understanding. For example, Emily at four

1

was described as being 'very shy' by a nursery teacher. At ten, Emily could reflect back on this and say, 'Mummy, I'm not so shy as I used to be, am I?'

Thus, we all have a sense of knowing ourselves. Some people are more sensitive to this than others. Some people may feel they need help to understand themselves, particularly when things go wrong. But overall, a recognition and knowledge of self exists in all of us, although understanding the theoretical reasons for how this works proves to be much more complicated.

The theoretical definition of self

Psychology and philosophy have recognised the concept of self since Descartes in the seventeenth century. His *cogito ergo sum* (I think, therefore I am) emphasised the centrality of self in the consciousness. There have been many elaborate discussions over what constitutes the self since then. What is unique about the self is its *reflexiveness*. Our perception of any other object in the world involves subject and object being different. It is only the perception of the self which includes a construct of both subject and object.

Many people have defined the self, but historically one of the most important definitions came from William James (1890) who viewed the self as a distinct entity and divided it up into three parts. These were the constituents (the material self, the social self, and the pure ego), the feelings and emotions which these arouse; and finally the actions which these prompt (such as self-seeking, as an expansion of the person's goals and self-preservation). This definition obviously makes clear that the notion of self is multifaceted and complex, and this is where some of the debate lies. Is it possible to have one superordinate statement to describe the self or is it too complicated to be summed up in this way?

Rosenberg (1979, p. 7) defined the self as 'the totality of the persons' thoughts and feelings having reference to him/herself as an object'. However, a subsequent description included various facets which were the incorporation of a self-image, the person's reaction to the self-image, the evaluation of that self-image (whether the person has a favourable or unfavourable view of self) and what Rosenberg describes as a behavioural predisposition; that is what the person is likely to do in response to his evaluation of himself.

Thus, there is something about the self which involves knowing, but also involves evaluation. We not only know ourselves, we evaluate ourselves too. Your understanding of yourself involves a description (being a student) but also an evaluation (a good student, or a mediocre one). These evaluations may be public evaluations such as your view of yourself as a student, but they may be more private and reflect your inner experience. You may view yourself as weak and inadequate as compared with other people. You may view yourself as better than most. How this evaluation is used in our everyday understanding of ourselves has been a cause for much psychological investigation.

The self-concept

Most of us have a notion of self-concept to such an extent that a lot of psychological research looks at the self-concept of people in certain situations without defining the theoretical underpinning of the self-concept in any formal way. What is now apparent from the literature is that theoretical models of self-concept can be polarised into two broad perspectives; those supporting the unidimensionality of the construct versus those supporting multidimensionality. The understanding of the unidimensional model is that it is made up of overlapping facets of information which are given equal weight. Thus there is a general self-concept composed of, for example, academic, social and physical factors. Alternatively the multidimensional model is composed of multiple facets each of which is independent of all other dimensions. According to various authors these develop independently as a consequence of daily experience. There is a lot of debate within the psychological literature about the validity of the two different types of models (Byrne 1996).

The self-concept and self-esteem

What is also frequently debated is the relationship between the self-concept and self-esteem. It has been suggested that the self-concept is the cognitive part of self-perception and self-esteem is the affective dimension. Self-esteem is often viewed as being composed of two basic psychological processes, that of the process of self-evaluation and that of self-worth. Self-evaluation includes the comparison of the self image with the ideal self, and the internalisation of society's judgement on the self. This distinction of actual versus ideal self is viewed as an important construct in the understanding of self-esteem and self-understanding. That is, individuals may hold a view about their actual self which differs from the view of the way they would like to be. The ideal self or 'possible self' can be viewed as a motivational function where the individual may pursue aspects of self which relate to the ideal. In general, problems begin if the individual feels powerless to pursue any aspects of the ideal and thus feels worthless. For example, an individual may have an ideal self view which incorporates 'self as successful employee'. If that individual fails to find meaningful work then the inclusion of this aspect in the view of self is invalidating and potentially detrimental to psychological health.

Self-worth is the feeling that the self is important and effective. A lot of work has been done on how the evaluative side of the self relates to the more descriptive aspects. For example, some aspects of the self may be more salient than others in certain situations. When at work, my view of self as an academic is unaffected by my view of self as a mother.

Self-esteem is the process of self-appraisal which is influenced by self-evaluation and arguably, by evaluation by others. It is viewed as being susceptible to internal and external influences and mostly perceived to be traitlike in much the same way as is intelligence. It is assumed to be consistent over time within individuals although it may be susceptible to variation. For example, Baumeister (1995) quotes an example of how people's momentary self-evaluations fluctuate in response to short-term events; thus the implication is that self-esteem changes somewhat after each flattering or degrading event but then returns to a stable baseline. Pelham and Swann (1989) evaluated the factors which contributed to the individual's global self-esteem and extrapolated the following three factors. That is, the role of affective experiences in determining feelings of positive or negative wellbeing, the individual's specific self-view and the way the individual 'frames' the self-view such as discrepancy between actual and ideal self. The discrepancy between actual and ideal self is often presented as a reason for depression. That is, the individual's self-view is so distant from their ideal self-view that they experience profound negative feelings. The individual feels so distant from how he or she would like to be that depression results. The role of early experience in determining the individual's self-worth is also emphasised. Care givers can impart feelings of self-worth to infants that can have long-term consequences and influence the way adults later see themselves.

In general, we believe that it is important to have high self-esteem. Low self-esteem is undesirable and research has linked it to loneliness, depression and social anxiety (Blascovich and Tomaka 1991). The difficulty with this as a theoretical concept is that it is hard to determine whether low self-esteem is a causative factor or whether it occurs as the result of other conditions. Poor economic situations and dependency on state benefits may cause low self-esteem as a response to the individual's situation. Various researchers have explored low self-esteem and attempted to find explanations for why this should occur. High self-esteem people are generally motivated towards self-enhancement, while low self-esteem people are guided by an overriding feeling of self-protection.

The self in society

Several authors have considered the self to result solely from social interaction whereas others have considered the interactionist model to be only a part. That is, the individual learns about self through the interactions with other people and importantly has the capacity to do this. The self is able to have an understanding which includes the perception of other people's perception of the self. This has been referred to as the 'looking-glass self' or is incorporated into the concept of 'reflected appraisals'. That is, the way that others see us (actual appraisals) influences the way we believe they see us (reflected appraisal). It has been suggested that the discrepancy between the way others see us and the way we believe they see us may account for problems in psychological wellbeing.

There is general agreement that our self-concept is influenced by our attempts to compare and contrast ourselves to significant people in our lives. Festinger (1954) developed the theory of social comparison which is the process by which we compare ourselves to others. This includes other people's abilities, opinions and beliefs. Festinger hypothesised that the individual's personal development included a drive or motivational force to make these comparisons.

If social interaction accounts for a substantial degree of the development of the self, then the development of the self in children will be affected by the quality of social interaction and the child's own capacity for that interaction. Self-concept development takes place alongside rapid general development and language expansion. However, if developmental problems exist, the potential to develop a strong sense of self must be put at risk.

Kelly's (1955) personal construct theory owes its origins to existentialism, but is frequently a theory attributed to both psychological and sociological texts. Kelly accounted for the individual's behaviour and personality by the means of a system of bipolar constructs, that is a construct system which allowed the individual to make sense of and interpret social and personal reality. The main thesis is that the individual is constantly experimenting with every moment of reality and the constructs serve as the means of bringing order to the experiments. The constructs allow the individual to predict, for example, ordinary everyday things, like if I sit down on this chair I am more or less certain that it will support me; through to more abstract issues like, because I am a responsible person I predict that I will be able to look after this group of children well (thus I have a set of constructs about chairs being safe supportive structures, and a set of constructs about myself as a responsible person). Construct systems can work independently of each other, be subsumed under each other or be networked together. Therefore the construct allows for a construct of self, and also has a means of describing self. Kelly accounted for the concept of self by defining core role constructs: 'Core constructs are those which govern a person's maintenance processes – that is, those by which he maintains his identity and his existence' (1955 p. 482).

What is important here is that the process of construing this stable sense of self is composed of feedback in many forms. So that within this definition Kelly allows for the individual's core self to contain his construction of himself, alongside his construction of how he believes other people see him and thus his construction of himself in a role in society. Winter (1992) in an extensive discussion of the clinical application of this theory, discusses the central importance of self-construing in a variety of clinical disorders such as people with neurotic disorders (Winter and Gourney 1987; Button 1990), agoraphobia (Lorenzini, Sassasoli and Rocchi 1988), problematic children (Jackson 1990) and people with anorexia (Button 1987).

Social cognition

From a social cognition position, the self-concept is one of many types of cognitive structure. Schema theory looks at general assumptions which individuals and how those assumptions affect the way they experience the world. Fiske and Taylor (1992, p. 13) define schema as 'a cognitive structure that represents one's general knowledge about a given concept or stimulus domain'. That is, the way in which we perceive things is affected by the cognitive structure which gives information to the incoming stimulus. Thus, there is a theoretical justification for self-schema; that is the knowledge developed over time about self which is used to guide every experience.

Self-efficacy is a theory of social cognition (Bandura 1977) which formed part of an overall theory about behavioural change. That is, the individual's belief about personal effectiveness is an important aspect of the self-concept and self-esteem. If an individual feels a sense of competence for an ability that is personally valued (e.g. the ability to speak in public when the individual views that as an important ability) then this will contribute to a feeling of high self-esteem. The theory states that behaviours are governed by a) outcome value (the importance of certain outcomes, or goals); b) outcome expectancies (expectations concerning the effectiveness of certain behavioural means in producing these outcomes; c) self-efficacy expectancy (judgements and expectations concerning behavioural skills and capabilities and the likelihood of being able to successfully implement certain courses of action).

Importantly, self-efficacy theory focuses on the more cognitive aspects of mastery and effectiveness rather than on feelings and needs. The fundamental understanding is that all aspects of behavioural or psychological change are dependent on the alteration of the individual's sense of personal competence. Four sources of information are recognised as being influential on self-efficacy, and these are performance or enactment experiences, vicarious experiences, verbal persuasion and emotional or physiological arousal. Performance experiences relate to information following attempts at completing a task, for example trying to lose weight, where the individual may experience a feeling of success after managing to control eating behaviour or a feeling of failure if he or she gives in to urges to eat high-fat food. Vicarious experiences relate to the observations that we make of individuals which we then use to affect our own behaviour; that is, where the observed person becomes a model for comparison. Verbal persuasion is viewed as less important than performance and vicarious experiences, but it has been shown to be affected by how trustworthy the individual perceives the persuader to be. Emotional or physiological arousal affects behaviour when the attempts at changing behaviour are associated with negative feelings, for example speaking attempts which cause poor reactions in the listener (as in the case of stuttering for example).

Another factor in this occurs around the value the individual places upon the particular skill. Thus, if the perceived competence of a *valued* ability is judged to be low then this will contribute to a feeling of low self-esteem (e.g. perceiving oneself as bad at public speaking but valuing that skill at the same time). Obviously, beliefs about self-competence will have a direct effect on the definition of the self. It has been argued that self-efficacy beliefs are more context specific than overall views of the self-concept. Thus, as an example, a communicatively impaired individual may have self-efficacy beliefs about making a telephone call which are neither affected by global self-concept nor comparisons with others. Self-efficacy theories have been shown to be important in the health context where self-efficacy can influence anxiety, depression and low self-esteem.

The developing self-concept

There is very little work which has looked at the self-perceptions of children with communicative disorder, but clearly the implications from the work with adults are that the child may have a developing self-concept in spite of limitations in talking about it. In asking children to describe themselves it does acknowledge some level of self-understanding. Questions about the personal self over time, and about the characteristics of the self, all imply a certain level of knowledge and understanding.

It would seem that in developing a self-concept the child has to gain the ability to look at self as an object. Piaget (1936/52) stated that the ability to decentre from one's own egotistical point of view occurs during the preoperational period of development between the ages of two and six. It is generally encompassed in the development of social learning in the child. Another milestone in the development of the self-concept is the child's ability to understand that people have stable and enduring psychological qualities. In the work on normal children Garcia Torres (1990) explored the development of self-descriptions in the context of play. In this study, younger children were found to describe themselves by physical attributes, while psychological traits appear only around the age of seven years. It was also found that the number of traits increase with age. Most five-year-old children were not able to describe themselves adequately, but by the age of eight children could usually describe themselves as part of a larger structure, such as the class or peer group. Certainly the rule appears to be that, in general, the older the child the greater the ability to describe self fully. Fox et al. (1996) noted that differences in personality style will ultimately affect child self-concept and contribute to continuity or discontinuity of styles over time. One of the other contributory factors is the child's development of a set of beliefs about standards of social behaviour in order that the child can use this as a basis for comparison. For example, in a class of seven-year-olds, individual children may build up a sense of self-understanding based on social rules about behaviour, with which they may use to compare themselves. Thus, child A may perceive himself as 'more naughty' than other children, while child B may perceive herself as 'better behaved' than other children.

What is also of interest is the notion that self-concept development is not merely an additive process. Hattie (1992) discusses the way in which adolescents are shown to understand themselves. In general they perceive themselves differently from younger children; they do not merely add on conceptions. Younger children are shown to use more concrete descriptions of self, whereas the adolescent prefers more abstract, interpersonal and psychological descriptions. It has been suggested that the use of the abstract conceptions parallels the advancement of cognitive skills and thus adolescents are much more able to incorporate concepts about themselves.

There is some evidence (Fox et al. 1996) that socially inhibited children as young as seven displayed poorer self-concepts and were more depressed and anxious than their sociable peers. If this result is found with children who were described as socially inhibited but who had no pathological disorder, then what are the implications here for the communicatively impaired child whose social relationships may well be scarred or distorted?

Meadow (1980) discusses the difference between children who are deaf and handicapped versus children with physical handicaps. In a relatively old study of polio victims (Davis 1963), it was found that physical appearance is the first realm in which the child takes significant notice of how he or she differs from other children. Surprisingly, Meadow (1980) quotes other studies which demonstrate the deaf child's more positive self-concept than that of the hearing child. The rationale for this is that the deaf child experiences a more limited educational context where any small achievement is rewarded by praise and thus the self-concept becomes focused on positive aspects. Obviously this needs to be explored further.

However, the same sort of result is found in the work by Kunnen (1990), who explored the perceived self-competencies of physically handicapped children and discovered that the handicapped children in this study showed less realism about their competencies than non-handicapped children. Flavell, Miller and Miller (1993) discuss the normal child's overestimation of abilities. This has been frequently observed in other studies. The authors suggest that children confuse the wish to be competent with the reality, or that they lack a mature concept of ability and so cannot compare themselves with it.

The role of language in the definition of self

Interest in how a person views, interprets and thinks about themselves in relation to the rest of the world assumes that the person has a language capacity to do this. Language is viewed as essential to function in a social life, to express functional aspects of everyday communication and to express higher order aspects of emotion and beliefs. The multifaceted role of language must play a critical part in the process of the self-concept, yet it is one which is relatively poorly explored.

Burns (1979) states that self-descriptions can only be reported in words. If people have a limited vocabulary (for a variety of reasons) does this mean that they will be unable to describe themselves accurately? Does an impoverished vocabulary indicate an impoverished view of self? This is still a theoretical question which we need to explore. Sabat and Harre (1992) present evidence for the persistence of self-identity into the last stages of Alzheimer's disease. They report that self can continue to exist provided the care givers do not position the individual as helpless and confused. Carr (unpublished) reports two right-hemisphere damaged people, JG and RM, who, in spite of major right-hemisphere communication difficulties, demonstrated awareness of change in their circumstances since their stroke. Brumfitt (1985) looked at good aphasic speakers and severely impaired aphasic people. When using a repertory grid approach, both groups were able to differentiate between elements of past, present and ideal self. Although there were limitations in this study partly because of the cognitive complexity of the task, there is sufficient evidence to acknowledge that a sense of self can be preserved even in the most impaired communicator.

Joanette, Lafond and Lecours (1993) briefly discuss the implications of defining self in aphasia. They quote the aphasic person who said, 'I no more have the word inside me than I do outside' (p. 36) and suggest that the generation of that thought is related to internal language which is related to the external communication. They discuss the notion that there may be a non-linguistic dimension to thought which, in keeping with work by Sokolov (1972) accounts for everyday functioning by a form of concrete thought which does not require an elaborate internal language to be maintained. Joanette, Lafond and Lecours suggest (without empirical evidence) that this is why the aphasic person may have a self-view in spite of the substantial linguistic problems.

The role of memory in the definition of self

Many authors have acknowledged that memory plays a part in the development and maintenance of the self-concept. So far, however, the exact role it plays has not been demonstrated. It has been suggested that the self is composed of autobiographical memories which allow us to construct an identity over time. This by implication assumes that, for the most part, the autobiographical memories rely on the long-term memory system. In the organisation of memory, there is a distinction made between episodic (autobiographical) and semantic (language and knowledge) memory (Tulving 1993). Arguably, this could also be distinguished by episodic memories being about the subjective reality of the self, and semantic memories representing objective reality. Of course there is overlap here but in general the personal memories that individuals rely on to make sense of themselves are thought to exist in the separate system of episodic memory. Evidence about the long-term memory function overall, however, has demonstrated that although the storage of memories may be permanent, the recall of it is certainly not faultless in people without handicap. It is further compromised in people with intellectual deficits, and this is particularly related to Alzheimer's disease (Bartlett 1932).

Tulving (1993) describes an exceptionally unusual investigation of self-knowledge of an amnesic individual, KC, who at the age of thirty suffered a severe closed head injury which left him with severe amnesia and personality change. Tulving makes the distinction between summary representations of traits in the semantic system, as compared with episodic memory which enables the individual to remember personally experienced events in a network of other personal events. Tulving uses the data from KC to show that, although semantic and episodic memory share many of the same features, semantic knowledge can be stored and retrieved independently of the episodic memory system. That is, episodic memory can enhance the workings of semantic memory.

KC had post-morbid intact IQ within the normal range, normal language comprehension and could read and write normally. There was no confusion and he had intact short-term memory. He had no long-term memory and could not recall a single thing that happened to him and thus had dense anterograde and retrograde amnesia. His personality was described as changing to being more withdrawn, less spontaneous and passive. In Tulving's experiment he was tested for knowledge of himself and his mother. He was asked to do this by rating himself and then his mother on 72 traits. Based on these responses a new 32 forced choice test was given on two separate occasions. The results from these two tests were compared with his mothers' ratings of him, and it was found that he agreed with his mother 73 per cent of the time. Also, the trait judgements he did for himself did not agree at all with his mothers' choices for the pre-morbid KC. Tulving suggests that this data shows that KC's self-knowledge of traits cannot be based on remembering behavioural events from his pre-morbid life. The importance of this study is that it suggests that trait judgements can be made without reference to trait relevant autobiographical episodes, and therefore that they can be held in the semantic memory. This clearly has implications for the role of semantic memory in the language impaired individual. We do not know, for example, how reliably the aphasic person could complete the trait judgement task. If the meaning of the word is to link in with a self-judgement and can be done purely by semantic memory as Tulving suggests, is it then implicit that the aphasic's self-report *has* to make use of autobiographical memory because the semantic memory system is so unreliable?

In a more qualitative way, Howitt et al. (1992) note the importance of Neisser's 'extended self' which relates to past self and the future anticipation of self. The implication is for a continuing life history which carries with it memories of past events which have helped to form the present notion of the self-concept. Horrocks and Jackson (1972) also note the importance of the self as containing the experiences of the past, present and expectations of the future.

Spinelli (1989) argues that although the basic facts about ourselves are stored in the long-term memory, our interpretation of these may change over time. For example, an event which may have felt disastrous in our early twenties may be viewed as an important learning experience when evaluated in our fifties. Thus by changing the status and meaning of an event the individual redefines the self.

How might this process work with someone with a communication problem such as aphasia? There is certainly no evidence to suggest that aphasic people cannot remember their past. But can they define it? If aphasic people have less access to the lexicon and therefore cannot define themselves in a meaningful way, are there implications for being aphasic which are as yet unrecognised?

Is it possible to assume that a core sense of self exists but which is less accessible via language in the aphasic person? This is a difficult question to answer, not only because of the complexity of the concept, but also because of the lack of measurement procedures available for aphasic people in this area.

How can we arrive at understanding the individual's self view?

Personality theory, social learning theory, social cognition and motivational theories have all contributed to the ways in which the concept of self is assessed or determined. In psychology there has been a substantial debate about the ways in which the self-concept is measured. Hattie (1992) describes all aspects of measuring and determining the self-concept and notes the dependance on the individual's inclination or ability to self-report. Burns (1979, p. 9) also notes that the relationship between self-concept and self-report is dependent on several factors. These are:

a) the clarity of the individual's awareness
b) the availability of adequate symbols for expression

c) the willingness of the individual to cooperate
d) social expectancy
e) the individual's feeling of personal adequacy
f) his feelings of freedom from threat.

With the communicatively impaired population, there is an obvious difficulty in ensuring clarity of awareness, certainly with some client groups, and
the availability of expressive symbols. Thus many of the formalised
approaches to evaluating the self are either too difficult to use or else have
not been properly evaluated. Almost all self-perception measures are
demonstrated to be suitable for normal speakers and the developmental
studies of these measures never include communicatively impaired groups.
However, this does not imply that all of the approaches are inappropriate.
There is no reason why many of these could not be developed and modified
to take account of the individual communicative differences.

Several of these approaches will be presented here for further reflection.
Semantic differentials are a very common procedure to use to evaluate the
self-concept. These require the respondent to rate self in relation to a
series of bipolar stimulus words (such as good–bad, happy–sad). Osgood,
Suci and Tannenbaum (1957) identified three basic dimensions that the
differential typically assessed: a) evaluation (good–bad, valuable–worthless); b) activity (fast–slow, active–passive); and c) potency (strong–weak,
large–small). Semantic differentials are frequently used in psychological
studies which require a self-descriptive measure.

Q sorts is a technique which uses statements about the self-concept on
cards. The most popular is the version by Butler and Haigh (1954) which
contains 100 self-referent items for indexing the self-concept. These are
required to be sorted into nine piles arranged on a continuum according
to the degree to which the individual claims they are characteristic of self.
It is also suggested that the individual completes several sorts under
different instructions, such as self-concept, spouse's self-concept and so
on. This approach is viewed as time consuming, but has been used in
research such as with Rogers (Rogers and Dymond 1954) in
psychotherapy.

The twenty statements test (Kuhn and McPartland 1954) asks for
twenty statements to the question 'Who am I?'. The answers are then
coded into four categories:

- category A includes physical attributes (the physical self)
- category B contains references to statements which are socially defined
  (the social self)
- category C are more abstract and describe styles of behaviour (the
  reflective self)
- category D refer to superordinate descriptions of the self, such as 'I'm a
  person who wants the best for everyone' (the oceanic self).

Unstructured and free response methods have been used in order to allow the respondent an opportunity to respond without the limitation of rating scales. The usual objection to this approach has been the difficulty in classifying the responses. However, the more recent developments in qualitative psychological approaches have shown that analysis of themes and a rigorous approach to developing a theory about the person's account has tightened the procedure sufficiently.

Use of Kelly's repertory grid technique has been applied to many conditions and to some communication disorders. It is used most commonly with people who have stuttering problems, but it has also been used with people who have aphasic problems (Brumfitt 1985). Many examples of repertory grid technique exist in the literature (Fransella 1972) and conform to the general rules set down by Kelly (1955) whereby the grid is composed of elements (self-descriptions, for example, past self, present self, future self, ideal self) and elicited constructs. The constructions that the individual places on personal experience are intended to permit an understanding of what is important to the individual and where there is potential for change.

Self-characterisation has also been used to explore the individual's self beliefs (Kelly 1955). It has been described as a means of helping the therapist 'enter the client's personal world' (Hayhow and Levy 1989, p. 23). The instructions for the self-characterisation are very specific.

> I want you to write a character sketch of ... just as if he/she were the principal character in a play. Write it as it might be written by a friend who knew him very intimately and very sympathetically, perhaps better than anyone ever could know him. Be sure to write it in the third person. For example, start out by saying '... is ...' (Kelly 1955, p. 323)

The individual is then required to write as much as possible and the characterisation is analysed by extrapolating specific themes and the significance of certain words or phrases which recur. Self-characterisations have been adapted by Jackson and Bannister (1985) for use with children between the ages of nine and thirteen years. The instructions have had to be modified.

> Tell me what sort of boy or girl X is. If you like I will be your secretary and write down what you say. Tell me about yourself as if you were being described by an imaginary friend who knows you and likes you and above all understands you very well. This person would be able to say what your character is and everything about you. Perhaps you could begin with, X is ... and say something important about yourself. Try to fill this page.

Jackson (1985) described categories for analysis of the children's characterisation and these include statements about self-esteem, non-psychological statements, psychological statements, personal history, conflict, insight, views of others and psychological cause and effect (these are presented in the exercises at the end of this chapter).

Some measures have been developed specifically to determine the level of self-esteem experienced by the individual. Rosenberg's (1965) self-esteem scale consists of ten statements, five of which are phrased in the positive direction with the other five in the negative direction. These are rated on a four-point scale ranging from strongly agree to strongly disagree. This scale has shown very acceptable reliability. As it focuses on a specific facet of the self the results derived have to be used alongside other measures if a broad, all-encompassing view of self is required.

It is important to note the inclusion of the need for adequate symbols for expression (Burns 1972). Almost all measures of self-concept presuppose the individual's ability first to understand the language, and interpret the language in a meaningful way in order to then indicate a verbal or written response to the stimulus.

The visual analogue self-esteem scale (VASES: Brumfitt and Sheeran 1999) has taken into account the communicative problems experienced by the aphasic speaker and provides a means of gaining a self-evaluation with the use of picture stimulus. The measure is based on pairs of pictures which represent concepts about the self (for example, dependent versus not dependent). The measure was developed because of the need to find a way of evaluating self-esteem where pictures and not simply words was essential and the rating procedure was simple enough for people with aphasic speakers to cope with. The aim of the measure was also to provide a scale which was short and easy to administer. The aphasic person has to rate each pair in relation to a view of self. Thus the task is to identify self-traits and gain an overall score that gives an indication of the level of self-esteem. It is suggested by the authors that this measure can be used in the acute stages of a patient's illness and subsequently for comparison later in the rehabilitation process.

In addition, Stern et al. (1997) have recently developed the visual analogue mood scales (VAMS) to measure mood in aphasia. Seven visual analogue mood scales were developed using vertical 100mm lines and simple, schematic faces to represent mood states. Each mood face was paired with a neutral face; the positioning of these pairs was constant; that is the neutral face was always at the top of the page and the mood face at the bottom. The 100mm vertical line connected the two faces. Vertical lines were chosen to take account of any visuospatial problems. The aim of this is to measure the newly aphasic speaker's mood in the initial stages post stroke.

Sutcliffe and Lincoln (1998) have recently developed the stroke aphasic depression questionnaire (SADQ) which aims to detect depressed mood on aphasic speakers in the community. The material does not use pictures but so far results have shown that it has good internal consistency and moderate validity and further research will be completed in the future.

The measure consists of ten items. All of these recent initiatives to find ways of understanding the self will have long term benefits for the aphasic speaker.

Some measures have been based on the use of drawing to represent self, but these are typically used for young children. Hattie (1992, p. 161) reports Wylie's review which stated that 'drawing yourself' has been used to:

a) assess perceptual-cognitive aspects of the drawer's body image
b) indicate emotional-evaluative reactions to the body
c) represent the drawer's self-concept or self evaluation other than cognates or feelings about the body.

Often there may be confusions about what the drawing task is really testing, although Hattie does report that drawing skill can be assessed at the same time as doing the drawing task to examine self-perception. There seems to be no similar test which is available for use with adults, although there must be a need given the range of disability which includes a major communicative disability. Possibly the communicative disability is so very often associated with motor or intellectual impairment that the use of drawing to represent self is too potentially inaccurate. However, this needs to be explored further.

Other approaches to evaluating children have been developed, for example by Byrne (1996, p. 69), who notes that any instrument for children must be designed so that it maintains the interest of the child, provides very concrete and specific descriptions of the question asked, uses a simple method of response and offsets the tendency towards socially desirable responding.

Before we discuss the implications of this for the person with a communication impairment we need to look at the predicament of the person with chronic disability and evaluate what is known about this.

The self and physical disability

Part of one's sense of self is the knowledge about one's physical being. Burns (1979) made a distinction between body image and body schema to convey the concept of the physical body which each individual possesses. The body schema is defined as the knowledge derived from the sensations of the body and the positions of its parts; the body image is an evaluated picture of the physical self. Clearly, there is a relationship between the two factors which are emphasised when the individual suffers a physical disability. Part of the individual's evaluation of the body includes the societal influences about what is attractive or not. How the individual incorporates physical disability into the self-image may be dependent on how visible the disability is. It is arguably easier to accept being disabled if the disability is on show all of the time, whereas disabilities that are not so obvious (such as aphasic speakers who are only 'disabled' when speaking) may be less easy. It has also been postulated that disabilities that form a central part of the self-image are more difficult for the individual to accept. The most frequently quoted example of this is the woman who suffers a mastectomy.

Kathy Charmaz has written extensively about the self-concept and the experience of the chronically ill person. She describes chronically ill adults observing their 'former self images crumbling away' (1983, p. 168) while there is no parallel evolution of a new sense of identity to incorporate their disability. She reports that the individuals suffer from having to lead restricted lives, the experience of social isolation, being discredited and burdening others. When discussing the discrediting of self she notes that this may result from the experiences in interacting with others and the loss of self which comes from the unmet expectations of the sick person. Charmaz reports detailed experiences with chronically ill people, such as her visit to the shops with a lady whose leg had been amputated. This lady chose not to wear a prosthesis and instead went in a wheelchair. While in a store, a little girl noticed the lady and cried out, 'Look mummy, that lady doesn't have a foot. Doesn't she look awful?' (p. 181). Charmaz notes that the lady experienced terrible distress and a discrediting of herself. Although she had been able to accept herself as disabled, she was forced to confront this in a deeply humiliating and painful way because of the observations of the little girl. Charmaz notes that the discrediting experience is not limited to those with obvious physical impairment, but that what does appear to be critical is the significance of the discrediting encounter. Thus the important issues are the perceived magnitude by the individual, the relative importance of who discredits, the situation in which discrediting takes place and the amount of repetition of discrediting events.

What may also affect this perception of self, according to Charmaz, is the way in which the chronically ill person may use visual evidence to further discredit the self. For example, women may report the distress they feel on observing the untidy and rarely cleaned house. When they are surrounded by examples of their present failing abilities, this only serves to increase the negative comparison between their past way of functioning and present way. As Charmaz says, 'they may devote much energy to apologising to others for their felt inadequacies. Indeed they may apologise for their very existence because they too share the assumption that in order to be fully human, one must be able to function fully' (p. 187).

Yet people clearly do come to terms with their condition and Charmaz has developed this further. Many people reported that experiencing chronic illness gave them a deeper understanding of life with new purposes and new values. This clearly was a process that the individual might or might not be able to work through. The success of this depended to some extent on the sort of supportive context the individual lived in but also the individual's capacity to value in a self which transcends the physical disability.

The self and communication impairment

One of the most well-investigated areas into this process comes from the knowledge base about stuttering. Unlike many other areas of understanding about communication impairment, there is a well-developed literature on the social psychology of the stutterer and the personal predicament. How the stutterer views himself in relation to his stuttering is fundamental to the impairment. Thus, the individualistic approach to therapy for stutterers is dependent on first examining the individual's personal understanding of self in the social context.

Of course, one of the difficulties in exploring the self-view of the communicatively impaired individual is that normally we rely on accurate and normal speech from the person who is self-describing. With this special population, whether it be aphasic speakers, dysarthric speakers or stuttering speakers, there is a fundamental difficulty in defining the self through language.

The person with a communication impairment

Self and identity in the stuttering individual

Fransella's (1972) application of personal construct theory to stuttering implicitly focuses on the individual's self-perception. How individual stutterers understand themselves in their social context is viewed as a critical part of their potential to respond to therapy. Also, their individual constructions of themselves and their listeners are used to moderate the therapeutic outcome. Fransella reviews the literature on the self-concept of stutterers and notes that various authors have viewed the self-concept to be critical in understanding the stuttering problem. Sheehan (1954) conceptualised stutterers as having a dichotomised self-concept. Stutterers know themselves as disabled speakers and find it hard to move towards a concept of self as fluent speakers. That is, stutterers may have a concept of what a fluent speaker is, but be unable to incorporate this into their own self-images. Fransella quotes Shearer (1961), who discussed the conflict between the 'horrible stuttering self and the free speaking normal self'. What has been of particular interest is Fransella's work, which looked at whether the stutterer actually viewed himself as a stutterer or not. Following analysis of the implications form of repertory grid (see Fransella 1972), it was found that stutterers do not necessarily construe themselves and other stutterers along the same construct dimensions; thus they do not see themselves as stutterers. Stutterers as a group are different from the individuals' construction of themselves as stutterers.

Subsequently the same sort of finding was produced by Kalinowski, Lerman and Watt (1987) where the perceptions of self and other in stutterers and non-stuttering groups was determined. Using a semantic differential scale the results indicated that stutterers' self-descriptions were remarkably similar to those of non-stutterers'. Also, non-stutterers described stutterers with a predominance of negative characteristics whereas stutterers described non-stutterers in a positive manner.

Of course, what needs to be investigated further is the reason why the stutterer does not view himself as the same as the rest of the stuttering population. Fransella quotes from another study (Fransella and Adams 1966) which explored the construing of an arsonist where a similar effect was found. That is, the arsonist did not view himself as like other arsonists (in spite of serving a prison sentence for arson).

Self and identity in the individual with an acquired communication impairment

What has had very little investigation in the past is the self-view of the aphasic speaker. Yet, if other conditions are used for comparison, the way the individual views their experience of the condition is important. For example, the self-perceptions of people with schizophrenia exist in the literature (McKay, McKenna and Laws 1996) and even bizarre conditions such as reduplicative paramnesia (Luzatti and Verga 1996). This certainly seems to indicate the importance of self-perception in even the most unusual condition.

One of the factors which has affected the limited amount of research in this area, has been the difficulty in discovering the impact on the individual with severe aphasia. Many aphasic speakers do not recover sufficient ability to communicate their experiences of the condition. Although various reports of the personal experience of aphasia exist in the literature, these are dependent on aphasic speakers who are extremely well recovered. Hodgins (1968, p. 65) recognised the impact immediately:

One's speech is very much part of one's personality. The fact that mine was once fluent and now was halting made me feel – conspicuous. I do not know the feelings of a person defaced by a burn or a scar, but I imagine them quite like the feelings I had, at first, about my tongue's new and unwelcome capacity.

Most of the reports emphasise the feelings of sadness, isolation and frustration, and a summary of these is presented by Joanette et al. (1993). Personal statements include the following (p. 30):

For over three months I was in a bleak gray black desert, barren, no sound, no colour ... insipid, endless, everything was dead.
I felt figuratively imprisoned in a tomb.
I'm not the same. But I thought I was the same. My life is a contradiction.
I noticed a change in me, I was another person, someone who was unable to express the little I knew, I was ashamed.

Clearly, these accounts are from people who have sufficient use of language to be able to express their reactions. There are many people with aphasia where the brain damage is so extreme that the articulation of feelings to this degree is impossible. Yet we have to use these personal accounts as evidence in the absence of other information.

Glozman and Tsyganok (1982) explored the personal responses to being aphasic. Their hypothesis was that aphasia would produce not only changes in communicative abilities, but also substantial changes to what they term 'self-assessment'. An experimental study was conducted to look at any potential disparities between the patient's self-assessment in the present as compared with pre-morbidly. Factors affecting the self-assessment such as age and sex were also explored. The polar profile (Rubinstein 1970) was used to determine the individual's self-assessment on a series of lines which contain sets of pairs of personality descriptions. The personality traits which were studied were grouped into four categories: emotional-volitional, activity, attitude towards others and communicativeness. Twenty-one aphasic people were studied; of these one subgroup of ten had anterior damage and eleven had posterior damage. A control group of spinal injured patients was used. No significant differences between present and past self-assessment were found in the control group, but 'pronounced' disparities in self-assessments were found on three scales for the aphasic people. These were, the emotional-volitional qualities, the activity and the communicativeness. This was higher in the group of people with anterior lesions as opposed to people with posterior lesions. The scale of traits characterising attitude towards others was relatively stable. No distinct correlation was found between changes in self-assessment and sex or age of the patients or severity of the speech defects.

The effects of rehabilitation on fourteen of the original patients were also studied at the end of a cycle of individual and group rehabilitation. In six people with anterior lesions a definitely improved self-assessment was demonstrated (i.e., a decrease in the extent of the discrepancies between self-assessment before and after the illness) on all the studied scales. In the posterior damaged group of eight patients, only five demonstrated improvement and the overall change was much smaller than the anterior group. Again, changes were not correlated with age or sex. Glozman and Tsyganok conclude that there is potential importance in looking at the relationship between personality changes and aphasia and how this may affect rehabilitation.

One of the most closely related areas to aphasia is that of the head-injured population. Work by Tyerman and Humphrey (1984) demonstrated changes in self-concept following head injury. Statements about anxiety and depression were common, and the people interviewed described themselves as significantly changed as the result of the head injury. Antonius, Beukelman and Reid (1995) also explored the personal understanding of people with acquired dysarthric problems and noted the difficulties of lack of personal insight in people with Parkinson's disease.

Children with communication impairment

Jones (1985) explored the self-concepts of handicapped children (ages 10–14) and compared them with those of non-handicapped children of the same age. They were compared on two measures, that of the Piers Harris children's self-concept scale (Piers and Harris 1984) and the human figure drawing test (Koppitz 1968). Within the handicapped group were a proportion (number not stated) of children who had speech and language handicaps. The results of the study indicated that the speech and language impaired children had significantly more negative self-concepts than non-handicapped students. They were found to experience high anxiety and negative feelings regarding their intelligence and school status and popularity. The emotional indicators determined by the human figure drawing test suggested immaturity, impulsivity, inadequacy, guilt over failure, withdrawal and anxiety. Jones noted the demonstrated significance of the self-concept in relation to academic achievement and concludes that enhancement of the self-concept in handicapped children could improve their overall educational potential.

Rinaldi (1996) reports the inner experiences of children with specific developmental language disability. Substantial problems are demonstrated as the result of the language involvement, such as difficulties with the interactive process of communication and difficulties understanding and using non-verbal communication to express or interpret emotion. What is important here is that Rinaldi reports the children as having particular problems in self-knowledge. It is noted that language-impaired children are often unable to answer or often give inaccurate information about themselves. Their perception of self as a friend appears to be unrealistic, often reporting that someone is a 'friend' when there is only a very weak relationship. Rinaldi notes that as the language-impaired child matures and reaches the ages of 9 to 10 years, the child becomes much more aware of relationship difficulties, at the same time the onus on communication and socialisation becomes greater. Rinaldi states, 'It is little wonder that low self-esteem appears a fairly common denominator for teenagers with specific language disorder' (p. 138).

Barrett and Jones (1996) note that children with learning difficulties may fail to reach the later stages of self-understanding because of cognitive difficulties. They discuss the implications of this for such children and note that various authors have suggested that the ability to construct internally consistent and experience related self-narratives has important links with the ability to form secure and intimate relationships. A relationship is recognised between self-awareness and the ability to be aware of the feelings and needs of others.

Clearly the relationship between self-concept and speech disability needs to be explored further in relation to the developing child. Do we have enough information about whether the child's communicative impairment actually impedes the development of the self-concept in the case, for example, of a child with specific language disabilities? If you have limited language how can you move towards self-understanding if you are without the words to describe yourself? Does the communicative impairment cause low self-esteem? Do the children place low value on themselves because they cannot talk adequately? In the case of children with non-fluency problems, do the children's sense of self become influenced by failed communicative attempts or does their poor self-image affect the success of their fluency in the first place?

Summary

There is a huge and compelling literature on the perception of self that could enhance our understanding of people who have communication problems. By informing ourselves about the effect upon self we would arm ourselves better to cope with therapeutic intervention because we could explore the relationship between therapeutic outcome and self-understanding.

How is a communication impairment experienced by the individual? We need to know, but there are difficulties ahead. There is the potential difficulty in getting to this understanding because of the problem itself. What an irony there is in this. An identified population who need better understanding because of an impairment which actually impedes our understanding of them.

In the next chapter we will look at the theory and application of attitudes and measurement and how this relates to our population.

Exercises

Analysis of self-characterisations

Here are some samples of self-characterisations from two children who have no disabilities.

Emily, aged 10
Emily hates cry babies. She doesn't like wearing skirts and dresses and girl stuff. She doesn't like goody goodies. She doesn't like show offs. Emily likes chocolate. She hates lentils. She's not very good at swimming (especially front crawl and back crawl). She doesn't like talking on the telephone. She likes animals a lot and she likes going on long walks if they are not boring but she likes climbing on rocks. She likes Blue Peter. She loves all her pets and she thinks Biscuit is the cuddliest. Perfume makes her cough a bit. She likes things that are funny but she hates history. Her favourite colour is blue. She likes marble cake a lot and hates it when people think they are really good and they never cry, but they cry all the time. She is good at playing the recorder but not so good at the violin.

Dulcie, aged 8

Dulcie is good at art. Dulcie is good at writing. Dulcie likes choosing her own clothes and she doesn't like it when Mummy chooses her clothes. Dulcie doesn't like meat apart from turkey and chicken. She likes fish fingers. Dulcie doesn't like dolls. Dulcie loves her mummy and daddy and Emily. Dulcie's favourite colour is yellow. She likes rabbits. She doesn't like it when her teeth scratch together. Dulcie likes travelling on aeroplanes. Dulcie likes Think and Solve. Dulcie likes the look of candle wax going down the candle and she likes fancy candles and colourful candles.

Categories suggested by Jackson for analysis of self-characterisation (1985)

Self-esteem	claims of competence or moral virtue
Non-psychological statements	behavioural statements, activities, physical descriptions
Psychological statements	feeling, thinking or construing
Personal history and future	past or possible referred to in psychological terms
Conflict	contradictory assertions
Insight	awareness of own short comings and resulting problems
Views of others	child refers to view of self that is taken by others
Psychological cause and effect	may be implicit or explicit

Here are some suggestions for interpreting the self-characterisation above.

Emily

Her self-descriptions show examples of both psychological and non-psychological statements, e.g. psychological: 'hates cry babies', she 'hates it when people think they are really good and they never cry but they cry all the time'; non-psychological: 'she likes chocolate'. Also, there are examples of insight: 'she's not very good at swimming'.

Dulcie

Dulcie's self-descriptions show both psychological and non-psychological statements, e.g. psychological: 'Dulcie loves her mummy and daddy and Emily'; non-psychological: 'Dulcie likes travelling on aeroplanes'. She shows insight: 'doesn't like it when mummy chooses her clothes'.

Overall, neither demonstrate examples of conflict or psychological cause and effect and this may be because of their young ages. However, even these small examples can show that it is possible to gain insight into what can be important in the self-understanding of young children.

Who are you?

On meeting a stranger you are required to give an account of who you are. Write down five terms which best describe yourself to another person.

Look at what you have written. Is this what you expected? Have you put anything which you need to reflect further on?

Recommended reading

Baumeister RF (1995) Self and identity; an introduction. In Tesser A (ed.). Advanced Social Psychology. McGraw Hill Inc.

Byrne B (1996) Measuring Self-concept Across the Life Span. Washington DC: American Psychological Association.

Rosenberg M (1965) Society and the Adolescent Self Image. Princeton NJ: Princeton University Press.

Chapter 2
Attitudes

Overview

From this chapter you will be able to:

- understand what we know about attitudes and the relevance of this to the way individuals function in society
- understand how attitudes can be measured
- develop insight into how attitudes can critically influence how the client responds to therapy and the way the therapist also responds.

Introduction

Imagine you meet for the first time a person – a man, say – with aphasia. If communication is extremely difficult you may have to develop an understanding of him by ways other than speech. What do you think about men? Insensitive, unreliable and dominant? Or perhaps needing to be looked after, emotionally impoverished and dependent? This man looks old. What do you believe about being old? That it is a time of decline, incoherence and poverty? Or a time for seeking new challenges, enjoying the twilight of the years and being more content? He is wearing an old jacket which smells of cigarettes. What do you think about people who smoke? People who wear old clothes?

Before you begin to work with this client your own beliefs and attitudes may have affected your judgement about him.

What are attitudes?

Attitudes are generally thought of as the evaluations which people hold of themselves, or of other people, objects and issues. You may have an attitude to chocolate – do you like it or dislike it? You may have an attitude to politicians, or capital punishment or surrogate mothers. All of these attitudes make up the composition of you as a person even though you may not be consciously aware of your attitude to something until it is challenged. Petty (1995) describes attitudes as being based on a) affect or feelings (such as deciding you do not like cigarettes because the smell makes you feel sick), b) cognitions or beliefs and knowledge (such as evaluating cigarettes based on your knowledge about their health risks), c) behaviours or actions (such as deciding you prefer smoke-free restaurants as you always go to that type) or d) some combination of these. Your attitude may be based on these factors but it may also have an impact on them. Petty (1995) gives the example of how a favourable attitude can cause you to

a) feel happy in the presence of someone you like (affective influence),
b) think of mostly positive characteristics when asked to consider a person's application for a job (cognitive influence), and
c) agree to loan the person lunch money when she forgets her purse (behavioural influence).

It has been most recently suggested that attitudes may be based on just one or two of the components. For example, some attitudes may be based on how the object makes us feel whereas other attitudes may be based on how the object makes us think. This has important implications for exploring what influences our change in attitude; is it the affective or cognitive basis of the attitude?

In a way an attitude enables the individual to make sense of the world quickly. You see a person who staggers along the road looking unkempt and dirty. You quickly decide that this person is to be avoided as he may be drunk, likely to attack you and potentially dangerous. Your attitudes may have developed as you were growing up (beware of strange men dear) or have been the result of your experience (learning to mix with many types of people while at University for example). Attitudes can reflect an individual person's ambivalence about something. That is, such as feeling wonderful when we eat a large bar of comforting chocolate, but also realising that this has a high fat value and may affect health and weight. For market researchers this is something of a problem. From the point of view of the market place it is essential to establish whether you are likely to be influenced more by the affective aspect (chocolate is nice) or the cognitive influence (chocolate is bad for you). That is, those people who are more likely to be affected by the emotional need to eat chocolate can be identified as high consumers of chocolate.

Understanding what attitudes are is important because it then allows us to move on and consider what can be done to change them. This has implications in the health context as well as in the market place.

Attitudes allow us to categorise our world quickly. An attitude towards an object may permit you to make a quick decision about what you perceive. So much of our reality is based on the continual influx of information which is provided by our senses and we need a way of understanding it. In a sense, an attitude acts as a sort of screening process; it permits us to relate new information to the information which we already possess. It can serve as a frame of reference that can save time by organising the new information into a previously organised set of information. The way in which we are motivated to hold certain attitudes is also important. It has been demonstrated that we are motivated to have certain attitudes because of the influence of the group in which we operate and the need to be approved of by the group. An individual is motivated to belong to a group, and this may be general, such as being female and so part of the wider group of women, or more specific, such as belonging to a group whose role is to hold and maintain certain attitudes for political or sociological reasons (such as belonging to the National Childbirth Trust and supporting breast feeding for all mothers, or supporting the return of hanging for capital offences in Great Britain).

Of course, it is not necessary for an attitude to be extreme. It is argued that the strength of an argument is affected by the factors which have contributed to the attitude formation. Many researchers indicate that attitudes may be formed in the developing child who is exposed to family members and their attitudes. The child is 'rewarded' for holding the same set of attitudes as his parents. Similarly the child is exposed to adult behaviours which may mean he unconsciously learns to hold the same attitudes as them. For example, the child may be out walking with his parents and come across an injured bird. Because the parents hold a set of attitudes about the importance of preserving wildlife, the child observes his parents taking the bird home to try to nurse it back to health. Thus the experience has facilitated his development of attitudes towards wildlife. As well as these influences, attitudes may develop because of direct experience. The individual can only hold an attitude towards eating food with garlic in when he or she has done so. Any other experience of garlic eating is second hand.

Holding certain attitudes may have very serious implications. Various authors have looked at the relationship between attitudes and behaviour; Emler (1993) discusses this relationship in the context of adolescence and reports that attitudes show the same pattern as behaviour. In the specific area of attitudes to law and authority and degree of involvement in delinquency, a very strong relationship has been demonstrated. That is, in adolescence attitudes to authority become less positive in association with developing delinquent behaviour. This is something of a contradiction when consideration is given to the ambivalence in attitude shown in certain contexts such as believing that smoking damages health but carrying on with the damaging behaviour. Clearly that situation is more complex, because in that context the individual's problem is associated with addictive behaviour too.

Not only is an understanding of attitudes important for the market place, law and criminal behaviour, it is also important for our understanding of health behaviours. Niven (1994) notes that many of the problems health care professionals experience with patients or clients stem from their attitudes. If patients have a carefree attitude to diet, for example, they may be less likely to heed warnings that their fatty diet is aggravating their existing heart condition. Individuals may keep appearing with the same health problem, despite attempts to persuade them to give up risky behaviours. The most frequently quoted example of this is smoking behaviour. Of course, the attitude towards a behaviour is only the first part of the problem. An individual may have a belief that smoking is unhealthy and be determined to give up, but the strongest negative attitude towards smoking may not be enough to facilitate behavioural change.

Attitude measurement

Having determined that attitudes are implicit, researchers have devoted great efforts to measuring them. How important is a certain attitude to the person's behaviour? Does the attitude stop a capacity to change? How is it possible to understand the individual's attitude? Is it only by asking the person? Sometimes the individual will not have a conscious awareness of what attitude he or she has to an object. Possibly the individual's behaviour may give more indications about attitude.

The most commonly recognised method for exploring attitudes is the attitude scale or questionnaire. Generally these consist of a series of statements about specific issues, with which respondents are required either to agree or disagree. This type of scale is known as the Likert scale, where a choice is presented between agreeing strongly with statements and disagreeing strongly with them. An example of this may be as follows.

Because of the BSE scare, it is now too dangerous to eat beef.
Agree strongly
Agree
Neither agree nor disagree
Disagree
Strongly disagree

I see no need to stop eating beef
Agree strongly
Agree
Neither agree nor disagree
Disagree
Strongly disagree

Respondents are required to indicate which statement best reflects their view. Usually scales include statements that represent a balanced view of all possible attitudes. To develop a scale like this, items have to be generated which are relevant to the subject which is to be explored. For in-depth investigation, the scale has to demonstrate that it is reliable and valid. Results need to be compared against other scales that may be measuring the same construct or else compared against scales that are different but associated with the construct. For example, a measure of self-esteem can be compared with a measure of depression as part of the process of validation of a scale. Various attitude scales are already in use in communicative disorder, such as the S24 scale which explores the attitude of stutterers to their communicative ability. This is based upon Erikson's 'S' scale (1969) which was subsequently reanalysed (Andrews and Cutler 1974), and reduced to 24 reliable statements about attitudes to stuttering. This scale was shown to distinguish between stutterers and non-stutterers in terms of attitudes towards communication. The sort of attitudinal statements which are included in the scale are: 'I talk easily with only a few people'; 'I wish I could say things as clearly as others do' and 'I do not mind speaking before a group'. The statistical work on this scale demonstrated a mean for stutterers as 19.22 (range 9–24, S.D. 4.24) and the mean for non-stutterers as 9.14 (range 1–21, S.D. 5.83). Thus, in this example, measurement of attitude can be used reliably to distinguish between speakers.

Stutterers' attitudes in more specific contexts can also be investigated. In a recent study, James, Cudd and Brumfitt (1998) explored stutterers' attitudes to using the telephone. Part of the survey included a Likert scale exploring the stutterers' personal responses to using the telephone. The survey revealed that stutterers tended to use the telephone less than non-stutterers and avoid it deliberately. Even if they did use the telephone, the stuttering population tended to be anxious particularly about making the telephone call as opposed to answering it. The survey included 223 people with stuttering problems and the scale is presented in Table 2.1.

Statements which were defined as relevant to the stutterer's predicament were used to form the basis for the questionnaire. Each statement is phrased to permit a response in the same direction; that is a strong agreement with the statement would produce a score of one. Thus the score can provide an interpretation of the respondent's attitude; a high score of 50 would demonstrate attitudes unlike that of most stutterers.

Measuring attitudes can provide basic information about an individual or group, but what is of additional importance is whether attitudes can change and what influences this.

Attitude change

There has been a lot of work done on how to change attitudes and why people's attitudes can change. For example, it has been shown that attitudes can change as the result of being given a new piece of information. In this way social change may take place as the result of attitude change. Our attitudes to eating beef have changed considerably in the last few years owing to the BSE crisis. Twenty years ago people would have believed they were eating luxury food which was good for them if given a plate of roast beef. Now a proportion of people will not eat beef because of the fear of disease. Many schools do not have beef on their school

Table 2.1. Stutterers' attitudes towards using the telephone

In this set of questions, we would like to find out a little about how you feel about using the telephone and any problems which you experience with it. The first part consists of a series of statements. Please indicate whether you agree or disagree by circling the appropriate number. If any of the statements are not relevant to you (for example, because you are not working), please leave that line unmarked.

	strongly agree	agree	neither agree nor disagree	disagree	strongly disagree
It is more difficult to speak to someone on the phone than face to face	1	2	3	4	5
It is more difficult to use the phone when someone else is in the room	1	2	3	4	5
It is easier to use the phone if there is a background distraction such as the radio or television	1	2	3	4	5
I feel very anxious when I know I have to make a telephone call	1	2	3	4	5
I feel very anxious when the phone rings and I know I have to answer it	1	2	3	4	5
I feel that my anxiety about the telephone affects my performance when using it	1	2	3	4	5
Concerns about using the telephone have affected my choice of career	1	2	3	4	5
Problems with using the telephone have affected my career development	1	2	3	4	5
Telephone use has been irrelevant to my career development	1	2	3	4	5
Therapy specifically designed to help people with telephoning problems would be useful	1	2	3	4	5

dinner menu. This societal shift has been brought about by information which has caused individuals to change their attitude to eating beef.

Niven (1994) notes that is much easier to change someone's attitude while it is being formed than to try to change it years later. This explains the reasons why so much effort is put into health education in children; the belief is that children who are brought up to believe that taking drugs damages health are less likely to succumb to them in later life. Religious beliefs too are often impressed upon children at a very young age in order to ensure their maintenance of religious practice in adulthood. Sometimes these strategies make sense, but often the attitudes developed in child-hood may prove to be invalidated in adulthood. For example, the child who is brought up to believe that people who marry stay happy forever may have to readjust an attitude to marriage should his or her own marriage break down.

Petty (1995) discusses the psychological process involved in making an attitude change. People are thought to engage in steps of a process in changing an attitude. These steps usually are attention, comprehension, learning, acceptance and retention of the message. Thus an individual may change an attitude based not only on receiving further information, but on that information being personally meaningful and easy to understand. Experimentally it has been shown that information which is difficult to understand is less likely to change the way an individual views something. In addition, people need to actively think and reflect upon the messages they receive. The way they evaluate the information has also been shown to influence whether they change their attitude. Thus understanding and remembering the information is critical, but only in combination with the individual's ability to reflect upon it. Indeed, the personal meaning has great influence. For example, if a politician promised larger salaries for speech and language therapists who obtained PhDs, those therapists who were about to register to do one would be more likely to take the view that this was a good idea, whereas those without one or without the wish to do one would be more likely to have a negative attitude towards the new policy.

However, as Petty points out, attitudes can be self-generated without new information being provided. In a series of experiments it was shown that reflective or enhanced thinking could cause an attitude shift. The individual can only do this with a firm knowledge base, but if that is the case the individual can re-evaluate attitudes by reflection.

Sometimes attitudes change as a result of increased understanding or knowledge about a specific context. For example, professional under-standing of people with communication impairments has significantly altered over the last decade. In the late 1960s the teaching about aphasic speakers who cried and were emotional was explained by the fact that the person suffered from emotional lability as a result of the brain damage.

The response by the professionals was to distance themselves from this behaviour and believe that the aphasic person had uncontrollable emotions because of the onslaught to the brain. There was never any suggestion that the aphasic person could be reacting naturally to a very traumatic event – that of losing the capacity to communicate. Nowadays, having an emotional response to becoming aphasic is seen as a natural event and indeed part of the process of coming to terms with the situation. Certainly some aphasic people are labile, but professional attitudes have permitted us to distinguish this from natural responses, and the approach to the aphasic person is much improved because of it.

Attitude change: therapeutic implications

Gregory (1979) discusses the importance of creating a change in attitude in people with a stuttering impairment who are attending for speech and language therapy. He described the ways in which attitudes could change during the course of therapy by the way the therapist interacts with the client (p. 20):

1 He searches out with the client certain attitudes as revealed by the client's verbal report.
2 He helps the client acquire new verbal labels, in other words, new terminology that helps extend his understanding of his attitudinal and overt behavioural responses.
3 He selectively rewards certain statements made by the client that he considers as indicating a change of thinking in the desired direction.
4 He makes certain interpretations that are appropriately timed.

Here the therapist implicitly changes the individual's attitude as part of the process of therapy. Additionally, if attitudinal change is deliberately set in motion then specific changes can be identified. Stewart (1982) explored the relationship between attitudes and behaviours in a group of eight people with stuttering problems who were on an eight-week group therapy programme. The programme was designed to include a pre-treatment measure of attitude to communication (S24) and a measure of attitude to and intention to use fluent 'technique' speech and non-fluent speech. Following a programme of therapy the results showed that stutterers with low attitude and intention to use their own speech scores and those with high attitudes and intentions to use technique speech showed considerably greater fluency gains than those subjects with high attitudes and intentions to use their own speech and those with low attitudes and intentions to use technique speech. Thus Stewart was able to demonstrate some useful predictors about therapy; that stutterers with positive attitudes towards using a technique and negative views of their own speech are most likely to achieve more success in therapy.

Stereotyping

Stereotypes are the simplified categories that we use to make sense of people. Although they represent simplifications of understanding they also permit the individual to understand people quickly as individuals or in groups. Some of the earliest work on stereotyping stems from attempts to understand racism and prejudice in America. The main features of stereotypes are that judgements are quickly made about the visual appearance of people (for example, race, sex, nationality) and that all members of that category or social grouping are attributed with possessing the same characteristics. Although stereotypes are inaccurate understandings of people, they are often represent some truth, which is also an explanation for why we still use stereotyping in spite of our increased understanding of society and the individual.

Blane (1997) refers to work which looks at stereotyping of social class. Blane argues that social groups can be simply divided into two: the 'middle class', which consists of people who earn monthly salaries in non-manual jobs, borrow money to buy their own homes and support the view that education is important; and the 'working class', which consists of people who earn weekly wages in manual jobs, rent homes and aim for their children to leave school as soon as possible in order for them to begin earning money. Clearly there are many people who do not fit neatly into this grouping, but many people do have a more or less good enough 'fit'.

Sexual stereotypes have been frequently exposed as a way of explaining behaviour in a simplified way. The stereotypical assumption is that the biological gender should explain most aspects of an individual's behaviour. That is, that men are biologically aggressive and competitive whereas women are passive and nurturing. One of the most frequently used stereotypes of women is that women are biologically more delicate and prone to illness. Hillier and Scambler (1997) refer to the assumption that women are products of their reproductive system and therefore all of the associated conditions – such as cystitis, pelvic pain, premenstrual tension, menopausal symptoms – have been viewed in the past as 'not real' illnesses. The same authors refer to work which found that in the treatment of 'women's complaints' in family planning clinics, patients whose symptoms could not be treated successfully or diagnosed were classed as 'neurotic', and those who could not find a contraceptive which was suitable were classed as 'unreasonable'. Much research into the effects of stereotyping women in health care situations has been completed and improvements to health care achieved because of it.

The ageing person is often affected by stereotyping. The stereotypical old person walks with a stoop, is hard of hearing, gets confused and may exist in a state of poverty reflecting how good things had been in earlier times. Of course, this is clearly an inaccurate representation of elderly people nowadays. Many are wealthy, satisfied with life and have been able to avoid many of the health problems associated with ageing. Many internationally famous people fit into the elderly class – the Queen, for example, and Margaret Thatcher, who was in the elderly age group for part of her time in office as Prime Minister of Great Britain. Snyder and Miene (1994) investigated the stereotyping of the elderly and noted the long history of research into the stereotyping of the elderly going back into the 1950s. In general, the research demonstrated that perceptions of the elderly were negative, relating to deterioration in physical capabilities, and in personality themes such as 'old fashioned', 'authoritarian' or 'worried and weak'. As Snyder and Miene point out, however, as a stereotypical group the elderly are unique in that all of us will become members of this group if we live to the age of 65 and above. As they state, 'The way in which we view older people now is, in a very real sense, a view of our own future selves' (p. 65). They comment that it is difficult to understand how society willingly maintains a negative stereotype of something most people will actually become. There appears to be no gain from maintaining this view, whereas developing a positive view of the elderly would facilitate a much more helpful transition into later life.

Horsley and Fitzgibbon (1987) investigated the presence of a stereotype of children who stutter based on previous research which indicated that there was evidence for negative stereotype of the stuttering personality. They asked clinicians, students clinicians and teachers to rate eight bipolar constructs on a 25 bipolar rating scale to determine whether negative stereotypes were extended to children who stuttered. The results confirmed that the stuttering stereotype did exist, particularly for school age stuttering boys, and that the strength of this result was unaffected by actual exposure to stuttering individuals. Of course, there are many questions about how such a negative stereotype might occur. Although there is evidence to show that responses to the act of stuttering are negative (Dalton and Hardcastle 1977), there is other work which shows that it is possible to have a negative stereotype of a stutterer without any acquaintance of someone with this problem. Thus, there appears to be something within this culture which perpetuates the stereotype and maintains it in the discourse of the social context.

As Horsley and Fitzgibbon (1987) state, it is by no means clear whether or not stereotypical beliefs on the part of a clinician will affect the quality of a therapeutic interaction. Clearly, we need to gain more understanding of the relationship between clinician attitude and course and outcome of therapy.

Cognitive dissonance theory

Festinger (1957, 1964) developed the theory of cognitive dissonance. The original theory suggested that behaviour could lead to changes in attitudes. If an individual holds two attitudes or beliefs which contradict each other, then this is known as cognitive dissonance. For example, the individual who enjoys eating chocolate (positive attitude towards this high-calorie food) but also believes that high calorie food may cause weight gain (positive attitude towards health) will feel cognitive dissonance, that is, discomfort at two conflicting beliefs. One way of dealing with this is to change one of those attitudes (or dissonant elements). The individual could come to believe that chocolate did not taste as pleasant as previously thought and thus dissonance would be reduced. Many experimental studies have been done testing out this theory, exploring how individuals may cope with the dissonance. Because behaviour is difficult to change it is argued that changing attitudes might more quickly result in less dissonance or discomfort. Another example of this could be the person with a stuttering impairment who believed that 'being the life and soul of the party was the only way to be popular' and at the same time holding a personal view that he was a hopeless speaker in a social situation. Clearly dissonance would occur here unless the individual could be helped to change one element and perhaps arrive at the belief that it was possible to be popular without having to be the centre of attention at a social gathering. Other strategies are possible too. One way of reducing dissonance would be for the person to minimise the importance of one of the cognitions. For example, if social situations were viewed as unimportant then the inconsistency would be less trouble to the individual. Additionally, there could be an attempt to generate other cognitions which would make the dissonant elements consistent with each other. For example, a belief of 'I'm the sort of person who prefers to stay silent in social situations because I am so interested in observing other people' could be helpful here. Many of these strategies are already in use in therapeutic situations, but it would be useful to explore the application of this further. In terms of coping with a communication impairment we would want to know how dissonant cognitions might be identified and what sort of programme of help could demonstrate effectiveness of this sort of intervention.

Attitudes to disability

We all have attitudes to people with disabilities and these attitudes may have developed from our childhood experiences, our personal experience of someone with disability, cultural influences and professional education. There is no doubt that British society's attitude to disability has been to stigmatise and exclude people with disability until a more insightful policy about disability was developed in the last decade or so. Much of the literature about disability refers to the theme of exclusion from society and how attitudes of society to disability have actually added difficulties to the existing reality of disability. The disabled person has had to cope with his or her own responses as well as those of society.

There is no doubt, however, that attitudes have changed over the last few decades. Possibly this is owing to influences from the media who publicise the plight of the disabled and also the influence of charitable groups who have done much to champion equal rights for those with disability. However, it is thought that attitudes which are negative and prejudiced often exist because of ignorance and lack of information about a condition. Thus, as more public information about disabilities became available, so too did the increase in insight occur.

Thomas (1978) discusses the construct of social distance which refers to the degree of intimacy at which an individual would be at ease with another. In an old study of people's attitudes towards different types of disability, Jones, Gottfried and Owens (1966) found that loss of a limb was deemed to be a less serious disability to accept in a friend than a stutter, and that the 94 people used in their study would prefer to have an amputated limb than a stutter. It is posited that interactional awkwardness is a factor in assessing social distance and that this is why those people had such negative attitudes to people with stuttering problems.

It has been suggested that attitudes to handicap are deeply embedded in our cultural groups. Thomas refers to social history literature which reports various rationales for disability. For example, at one time children were deemed to be born disabled because of the misconduct of parents, or witchcraft. This, of course, led to the concealment of children with deformities and caused much of the social stigma that still exists today. The handicapped were of the lowest social order and thus had no rights to seek or claim help. In societies where being able to hunt for food was critical, the disabled were seen as economic liabilities; there is a clear relationship between attitudes to disability and a society's economic wealth. Thomas refers to work in the United States, Columbia and Peru and notes that there were progressively more positive attitudes to disability the more the economic status of the country improved. Although our attitudes to the disabled are so much more positive nowadays, it is important to recognise that these views have developed because of the relative wealth of our country.

In addition to cultural and economic factors, the political participation of disabled people had been criticised. Oliver and Zarb (1997) discuss the practical difficulties of the disabled person attempting to obtain a political voice in society. In one study (Fry 1987) it was found that many disabled people did not appear on the electoral register. Some blind and deaf people had no means of understanding the information on election choices, and the access problems to voting stations made it impossible for them to attend. Oliver argues that this failure to recognise the difficulties in participation has affected the quality of representation for the disabled. Thus, although attitudes have improved, there is still room for further enhancement of the rights of disabled people.

It is particularly important that medical clinicians are aware of detrimental attitudes towards people in their care. Garrett (1992), for example, reports that this may affect the diagnosis and management of people with aphasia. That is, a clinician who views elderly people as being 'slow' at communication may miss the sensitive diagnosis of aphasia.

Attitudes to communication disorder

Jordan and Kaiser (1996) refer to the fact that aphasic speakers are disabled even further by the attitudes that other people hold towards them. They argue that attitudes take on an added importance in relation to aphasia because language serves to convey attitudes as well as being the core aspect to the impairment. Thus, the potential for enabling people to change their attitude to aphasia is debilitated by the aphasic person's incapacity to represent him or herself. In addition, the aphasic speaker can only be seen as a disabled person when he or she attempts to speak, and thus the difficulty is well hidden. This makes it more difficult for people to form strong beliefs as they might do about someone who was in a wheel-chair. Jordan and Kaiser refer to Block and Yuker's statement: 'The most rejected persons are those with the most non-normal appearance or behaviour which may be hard to ignore. Thus facial disfigurement, brain damage involving strange speech patterns or strange gait are hard for people to adjust to' (Block and Yuker 1989, p.2; Jordan and Kaiser 1996, p. 163).

Attitudes to deaf people

In a study also referred to in Chapter 4, Gregory, Bishop and Sheldon (1995) explored the experiences of families of deaf children as a follow up to a study undertaken 18 years previously. The families were asked to reflect on the attitudes of other people to the deaf child. In the first study the parents had reported a general lack of understanding of deafness, but as the child had grown up much of this had improved. The explanation was that as the child became more mature the deafness was not such a dominant issue, and that attitudes towards deafness had slightly improved with society's increased knowledge about disability and handicap. The types of attitudes which were reported related to apathy and lack of under-standing. In particular, the medical profession was described as having poor awareness, always expecting parents to attend with their children (and, of course, still when they were adolescents) and expecting the parent to talk for their son or daughter. Hospital staff also were viewed as having a insensitive attitude. A particular concern for deaf young people was the negative attitude from employment situations, work training schemes and other interactions where professionals were employed to help young people gain employment but had no special insight into the predicament of the deaf person.

The attitude of a person with a communication impairment

The person with a stuttering impairment

> Speech Pathology appears to have largely neglected the numerous discussions in social psychology regarding the nature and role attitude plays in respect to behaviour. (Stewart 1996, p. 447)

Most of the work on attitudes and communication impairment stems from the American influence on stuttering. The stutterer's view of his or her speech and other people has always been considered a core part of the syndrome and thus has deserved substantial attention from both clinicians and researchers. Indeed, traditional therapy has involved examining and modifying attitudinal domains in order to make changes to speech patterns. The stutterer who has developed maladaptive beliefs about himself as a speaker may need to be offered therapy which will permit him to re-evaluate his speech and the way he presents himself. Watson (1995) reports the considerable interest in this area and the support for attending to covert aspects of stuttering as part of the therapeutic process. Various papers have explored the relationship between stuttering and attitudes and according to Watson, focused on three primary areas: a) examining attitude shifts post therapy; b) determining the influence of attitude changes upon maintenance of acquired speech patterns; c) evaluating the prognostic value of pre-therapy attitude assessment. What is important in this summary of research is that it mostly supports the view that there is an association between attitudes and stuttering behaviours. Subsequently, Watson has developed an inventory of communication attitudes (Watson 1988) from which results have shown that some adults who stutter have communication attitudes that are very much like adults who do not stutter, whereas some have attitudes very different from non-stuttering adults.

Stewart (1982, 1987) has made an extensive contribution to our understanding of attitudes and the role these play in the plight of the stutterer, particularly in relation to the stutterer's response to therapy. In a two-year follow-up study of 15 adult stutterers, fluency levels and attitude to fluent speech were evaluated. At the end of the study, significant changes were noted in the speech of the group of subjects.

Some change in attitude did take place during the programme. Interestingly, the attitude of group members to their own speech showed no evidence of modification, but what was most significant was the attitude of individuals to the use of a fluency technique and willingness to employ it in preference to non-fluent speech.

Silverman (1980) examined the communication attitudes of women who stuttered using the S24 attitudes to communication scale (Andrews and Cutler 1974). This was originally developed on male stutterers and the Silverman was interested to see if the responses were the same from female stutterers. Interestingly, scores from ten female stutterers, ten female non-stutterers and ten male stutterers demonstrated that differentiation from female stutterer to female non-stutterer could be made, as well as female stutterer to male stutterer. Silverman concluded that efforts in therapy towards normalisation of communication attitudes should be based, in part, upon the recognition of sex differences in human communication.

Attitudes of young stutterers

Research into the attitudes of young children to a stuttering problem has been scarce. Historically this may have been owing to the belief that young children should not have attention drawn to their stuttering difficulties in case this exacerbated the problem. The communication attitude (CAT) test (Brutten and Dunham 1989) was developed to measure the communicative attitudes of school-aged children. In the normalisation study, 518 non-stutterers were sampled and results indicated that these fluent speakers had minimal negative attitudes towards speech. Comparing stutterers and non-stutterers, DeNil, Brutten and Claeys (1986) found significant group and age differences within a Belgian sample; not only did the clinically diagnosed stutterers demonstrate more negative communication attitudes than the non-stutterers, but this difference was evident even among 7-year-olds. Of particular interest here is that children with developing stuttering difficulties may develop associated negative attitudes towards their speech at an early age.

Using the CAT test, DeNil and Brutten (1990) assessed the attitudes of other speech impaired children, who would also have potentially encountered negative communication experiences. The groups were: children with stuttering difficulties, voice disordered children, articulation disordered children and normal speaking children with mean group ages of 10.3, 10.5, 8.8 and 10.7 respectively. No significant differences in attitudes were found between the stutterers and voice disordered subjects, or between the articulation disorders and the control group. However, these latter two groups demonstrated fewer negative attitudes to do with communication than did either stutterers or voice disordered children.

Attitudes in other communication disorders

Myers and St Louis (1992), in a comprehensive book about cluttering difficulties, reported the distinction usually made between stutterers and clutterers about attitude to speaking. Generally, the stated view is that stutterers will have a fearful attitude to speaking, whereas clutterers will be careless about their speech. Indeed, this is a diagnostic criteria. Interestingly, Daly (1992), in a discussion of therapy for clutterers in the same book, reports the lack of clinical evidence for this reported phenomena. According to Daly almost all clutterers do care about their speaking ability. In an unpublished study, Wiles, Brumfitt and Cowell

(1997) found that a 32-year-old man, CR, had memories of choosing not to speak as a child because he was afraid of looking 'stupid'. CR was a clutterer with significant dyslexic problems, all of which remained undiagnosed until he left school because his behaviour was attributed to hyperactivity and 'low intelligence'. There is comparatively little experimental work on the area of beliefs about speech and self as a speaker with the cluttering population, but it is clearly worth pursuing.

Attitudes to using the telephone

Using the telephone is a very special type of communication and is normally attributed to the range of problems someone with a stuttering difficulty experiences. As shown in Table 2.1, in a recent survey by James, Brumfitt and Cudd (1998), over 200 people with stuttering problems reported specific difficulties with the telephone. Notably, the key attitude was that using the telephone was to be avoided if possible. The survey demonstrated that avoidance is more pronounced for making than for receiving telephone calls. Although a small percentage of the overall sample, it was interesting to see that 12.6 per cent of stutterers always used alternatives to telephoning because their attitude was that it was too difficult.

Dysarthric speakers

Work with dysarthric speakers has generated more acknowledgement of context and attitudinal factors. Antonius et al. (1996) refer to models of chronic disability in relation to the framework developed by the World Health Organisation (WHO 1992). This framework referred to four levels: the pathology level, which is the neurological diagnosis; the impairment level, described as 'loss and or abnormality of mental, emotional, physiological or anatomical structure or function'; the functional limitation level, which is defined as the inability to perform an activity within the normal range; and finally the inability to perform socially defined activities and roles within a social or physical environment. Speakers with Parkinson's disease have been found to be poor at appreciating the extent of their communication problems, and thus several studies have looked at their interpretation of different situations. Interestingly, in the study by Antonius et al. there was very little difference perceived between the six situational domains described in the study. These situation differences were: partner familiarity, size of audience, demand for intelligibility, demand for speed, emotional load and environmental adversity.

Aphasic speakers

Brumfitt and Sheeran (1997) reported the results of an intervention group for aphasic speakers. Unlike the dysarthric speakers, the raw scores give an indication that the aphasic speakers were making distinctions between situations in much the same way as stutterers. MW for example, on the Reactions to speech situations questionnaire (Williams 1963) at Time 1, reported very positive feelings about talking with a good friend, giving her name over the telephone, saying hello to a friend going by and talking to a friend about a personal problem. In contrast, she viewed some situations as being ones she would choose to avoid and disliked very much, such as telephoning to ask a price or fare, disagreeing with a friend, phoning to make an appointment or arrange a meeting place, and participating in a meeting. Although the analyses of the reactions to situations was not completed in the same way as the Antonius study, the data does set up questions about the capacity for insight and possible differences between Parkinson's disease speakers and aphasic people. Certainly of the aphasic people used in this study, they were able to demonstrate differences between their perception of situations, although this is such a small group it would be difficult to generalise it.

Rollin (1987) discusses the importance of attitudes to therapy in people with aphasia. The patient, according to Rollin, may have an 'unbending' attitude which may be counterproductive. Self-effacement, expressions of futility and resistance to practising at home may make the process of therapy very difficult indeed. Here Rollin advocates the use of therapeutic time to work on creating attitude change, because there is little likely of successful outcome without a positive attitude from the patient.

Attitudes to ageing

There is evidence to suggest that social attitudes to the elderly can influence cultural and individual responses to being old. Various authors have suggested that prejudice towards the elderly can cause more of a problem to the old person than the reality of increasing years and physical change (Slater 1984). Negative and inaccurate beliefs about being old have influenced the way in which society deals with the elderly. Typically, the view of the old person as hobbling about in a state of confusion and living in poverty persists, regardless of the many people who reach retirement age and are able to live productive and satisfying lives. Slater refers to Palmore's (1977) 'short facts on ageing' quiz, which tests beliefs about the elderly. The quiz asks makes statements such as 'Aged drivers have fewer accidents per person than drivers under the age of 65', and respondents are required to agree or disagree with this statement and others like it. Slater notes that the total score for correct beliefs is 20 and that first-year psychology students frequently score as low as 3 or 4.

Whether social attitudes can directly affect the 'decline' of the elderly person – and, in particular, cognition – is yet to be proven. However, there are certainly strong indications that it is difficult to maintain a positive psychological state if the individual is viewed as incompetent in some way.

Coleman (1993) notes that in an institutional setting competent behaviour can be undermined by attitudes of staff working in the institutions. It has been shown that even minor interventions can alter a situation; such as giving people more control over what is happening to them. Studies which have been well controlled have demonstrated improvements in mental alertness and increased involvement in activities where residents have been encouraged to take initiatives for themselves.

Summary

If attitudes affect general behaviour and more specifically professional behaviour, it is important to build this awareness into all that we undertake in professional intervention. The person who attends for help in the speech and language therapy context could be viewed as a summation of attitudes. Attitudes to the impairment, to other people, to having therapy and to you as a professional. You also have attitudes towards all aspects of your life, the patient, the type of impairment the patient has and your attitude towards different approches in therapy. If attitudes thus affect general behaviour and more specifically professional behaviour, it is important to build this awareness into all that we undertake in professional intervention. Exploring these attitudes can be a useful starting point for therapeutic intervention in many contexts and indeed it may be argued that failing to explore attitudes may delay or damage successful outcome in therapy.

In the next chapter we look at life transitions and how an understanding of this may help our client with communication impairment.

Exercise

Consider your answer to the following questions which are intended to draw out your attitudes to academic work, based on the understanding that attitudes are composed of how the object makes you feel, what your cognitions are about it, and how you behave.

1 What does doing a piece of academic work make you feel like?
2 Is doing academic work good for the individual?
3 Did you spend any time during the last weekend doing academic work?

Reflect on your conclusions.

Recommended reading

Horsley IA and Fitzgibbon CT (1987) Stuttering children: an investigation of a stereotype. BJDC 22(1): 19–37.

Petty RE (1995) Attitude change. In Tesser A (ed) Advanced Social Psychology. New York: McGraw Hill.

Stewart T (1987) Positive attitude to fluency: a group therapy programme. In Levy C (ed.) Stuttering Therapies: Practical Approaches. London: Croom Helm.

Stewart T (1996) A further application of the Fishbein and Ajzen model to therapy for adult stammerers. EJDC 31(4): 445–65.

Chapter 3
Life Transitions

Overview

This chapter will enable you to:

- gain a knowledge base about life transitions
- understand how this has been applied in speech and language therapy
- consider the ways in which this understanding could be applied further in clinical work.

Introduction

The 65-year-old man who has suffered a stroke is terribly distressed when you meet him for the first time. He has a small degree of right-sided paralysis and some communication problems and he is emotional and confused about his situation. In order to help, you begin to talk to him about his life and how he spent his time. Soon you begin to realise that not only had he suffered a sudden stroke, he had also just retired from his work as a company director and his eldest daughter had gone to live in Australia.

Sudden illness can affect us all at any stage of our life. But other difficult events may occur as the result of maturing, getting older, reaching a certain age and so on. This gentleman's distress was not only about his illness; it was about the separation from his daughter, and his retirement and loss of his previous lifestyle.

How might this knowledge affect what you do to help him?

Developmental aspects

Until recently, psychological development focused almost exclusively on the child. When a child reached maturity it was almost implicit that development ceased or at least remained steady. Now our understanding of people lets us recognise that development is happening all of the time. The individual grows and matures in a physical sense and accumulates psychological maturity alongside. This is generally known as 'life span' development and is an increasingly researched area in psychology. It is concerned with the explanation of the developmental processes involved in a person's life from conception to death. These developmental stages are influenced by physical 'norms', such as when the individual learns to walk and talk, but also by social and cultural expectations. Thus physical and cognitive maturity determines the point at which a child enters nursery school, but also our cultural expectation that the age of three or four is an appropriate time to begin to learn preschool skills. Similarly our expectations about leaving home or retiring are partly based on cultural and social norms and partly based on physical changes. Any sort of non-conforming behaviour tends to generate criticism and concern by society. For example, carrying on past the age of 65 in a career is generally viewed as unusual and cause for comment.

Erikson (1980) described eight stages of development used to define life transitions. Life transition is a construct used to describe times of change in the development during an individual's life. The transition is seen as something which can influence large areas of the life structure.

Erikson described eight stages of development which the individual moves through naturally. The interpretation is psychological; that is, not Freudian, but largely about everyday dealings in real life. Erikson's concern was with how the self deals with the social world. Thus the structure of thinking centres around the notion that the individual is born not fully formed in a psychological sense. As the individual matures, psychological maturity is reached by a series of different stages which culminate in a fully mature person. From Erikson's perspective, each stage represents a 'crisis' from which the individual is required to negotiate his or her way forward to the next stage. Failing to negotiate the stage may result in maladaptive development. Thus the emphasis is on the transitional aspect of development and whether the individual can successfully move from phase to phase.

The stages are spread throughout a person's life, with four occurring in childhood, one in adolescence and three in adulthood.

Stage 1 – basic trust versus mistrust (birth to one year). The importance of the mother/care giver relationship is highlighted at this stage and the success of the relationship will affect subsequent stages in the life cycle.

Stage 2 – autonomy versus shame and doubt (1–3 years). The child needs to develop confidence and independence. The parents play a crucial role here. The negative side of this is self-doubt and shame about perceived poor abilities.

Stage 3 – initiative versus guilt (3–6 years). Initiative results in the child going too far; he or she oversteps the mark. This stage relates to the context of parental control where the difficulty lies in how much the parent attempts to curb the child's natural initiative. Too much control can, according to Erikson, lead to guilt and a failure to achieve independence.

Stage 4 – industry versus authority (7–11 years) Here the child develops skills at school, and this can lead to the child feeling competent and confident providing the skills are achieved. The problem with this stage lies in the child who fails to achieve the skills and then is unable to move successfully into the next transition stage.

Stage 5 – identity versus role confusion (12–18 years). Here the adolescent struggles to develop a sense of identity during this intense stage of physical change. The crisis of identity is resolved when an integrated sense of self emerges and the adolescent achieves some self-knowledge.

Stage 6 – intimacy versus isolation (young adulthood). Here it is critical that an integrated identity emerges from Stage 5. Erikson takes the view that psychological intimacy can only be possible if Stage 5 has been a successful transition. The individual must be able to trust another person sufficiently to give him or herself to another. The critical issue is whether the individual becomes isolated and without close relationships.

Stage 7 – generativity versus stagnation (middle adulthood). Here the issues change and the individual is concerned with interests in the next generation, considering the future in general terms, and an increasing awareness of the quality of life and how it might be bettered.

Stage 8 – integrity versus despair (late adulthood, around retirement age). If the previous stages have been negotiated successfully then a sense of integrity will have emerged. Here the individual has to show acceptance of life and will be able to approach death without fear. The crisis focuses on whether the individual can now reflect on life and believe it to have been meaningful.

One of the most critical aspects of Erikson's theory relates to the successful move through each stage. The failure to proceed through each transitional stage is an explanation for why individual maladaptive behaviour takes place. For example, antisocial behaviour is attributed to failure to proceed normally through the critical childhood stages. Clearly, the child with significant communication impairments may have potentially more complex challenges to face moving from Stage 1 to Stage 4 of maturity and it is this area with which we may need to concern ourselves further.

Life events

Life events describe the experiences we all have which may be significant enough to cause a change in our lives. The events may be either positive or negative, but the critical aspect is that they cause change. Often a life event may cause psychological or physical problems because the stress of experiencing it may disrupt the individual's normal functioning. Clearly there is a difference between life events and life transitions in that everyone experiences life transitions as a developmental feature of life. Almost all of us (unless impaired by handicap) achieve physical maturity at around the age of 11 years and experience the psychological changes associated with this. However, the experience of what psychologists call life events is not necessarily a part of general development. Some people may experience the death of a spouse, while others do not. Some people experience divorce or separation while others do not.

A great deal of psychological research has been done on the definition of life events and much of this is attributed to Holmes and Rahe (1967) who in the 1960s developed a scale to measure the impact of life events. A large sample of people were asked to rate the amount of adjustment that each life event would require. Based on the item analysis of these, a social readjustment rating scale was developed which allocated 100 life change units to the death of a spouse and went down through all the major events to a value of 11 for minor violations of the law. The five most critical life events were: death of spouse, divorce, marital separation, a jail term, and death of a close family member. Of course, some life events can be defined more easily as one event than others. 'Trouble with the boss' (value = 20) is an event which may occur over time and be much less easy to attribute than death, which is obviously unambiguous. Frequently, too, people may attribute all sorts of difficulties to one life event such as bereavement, when it may actually be an unrelated event. For example, stress brought on by the death of a spouse may have no connection at all to the sudden need for the roof to be repaired, but because of the bereavement process the two events may be seen as connected in some way. The widow then perceives the death of her husband to be responsible for all the changes in her life.

Nelson Jones (1986) describes 'illustrative stressors which may contribute to a crisis'. These are descriptive and not the result of item analysis as is the work by Holmes and Rahe, but again there is clear emphasis on events which may cause a personal crisis for the individual and affect his or her progress through life. Nelson Jones divides the stressors into marriage and family aspects, such as living in a state of continuous marital conflict or death of spouse; occupational/educational groupings, which include reorganisation at work and public speaking difficulties; adverse social conditions, which include poverty and being subjected to racial discrimination; bodily harm, which refers to being battered by a spouse or drug abuse; and what is described as 'intrapersonal', which relates to problems including diagnosed psychiatric disorder and also generalised loss of meaning in life. All of these stressors can affect progress through life and the responses to any of these events, whether described using the stressor terminology or the social readjustment terminology, can have major implications for the way in which an individual moves through the normal transitional life stages.

In relation to our discussion here, every person with a communication impairment may also be coping with the communication problem in the context of other significant events. For example, a person with a stuttering problem can also be going through a divorce, expecting a baby, losing or gaining a job. Any of these life events may overrule the feelings the individual has about the communication handicap or influence the way the individual perceives his or her difficulties. For example, a person with a stuttering problem may attribute his divorce to the communication handicap ('If I could speak better then I would not be getting divorced'), or the loss of a job to the same cause. The mother with a learning disabled child attributes the slow development of her child to the death of her parents ('I just couldn't give him enough attention when I was looking after my sick parents, and now he cannot cope with school').

All of this discussion on life events also begs the question, does going through the experience of therapy in order to remediate a communication disorder cause a life event? Suffering a stroke and losing communicative ability does cause a major life event and discussion on this will come later, but coming for therapy for a stuttering difficulty may also come into this category. Some individuals with stuttering difficulties may suddenly gain insight through the process of the therapy. The covert behaviours used to hide the stuttering difficulty may through therapy now appear pointless to the individual and the value of confronting these covert behaviours, facing up to avoidance strategies and being open about stuttering may have such momentous meaning in the therapeutic programme that therapy itself may become a life event to be categorised alongside the others described here.

The small child

The preschool child has to experience all sorts of developmental changes which occur as part of psychological transition. Development is necessary to make sure the child learns security with one or two caretakers but is then able to move on and learns to trust other people too. In this way the child learns to adapt to different forms of child care and nursery education. As the child progresses through nursery towards more formal schooling, the challenges increase and the child learns to become more and more independent.

For the child with special needs this may be a more difficult transition. In a survey of deaf young people and their families (Gregory et al. 1995), the parents could recall the traumatic time their deaf children had on entering school. One mother explained that her child had such limited language it was impossible to explain to her where she was going. Because of the arrangements for transporting deaf children to a special school, the child was taken in a taxi without parents, unable to understand what was happening to her. As the authors note, parents of hearing children can help in a stage of transition because they can prepare their child for what is about to happen; they can talk about what it will be like at school and how the day will be spent, for example.

Deaf children have been frequently expected to cope with full-time education earlier than others. Some of the children in this study began at the age of three without any capacity to understand what was happening to them. Some of them were even sent to boarding school at this young age because there were no facilities for deaf children in the nearby locality. The parents talk of their 'hearts breaking' at the whole experience and feeling powerless to do anything about it. Apart from the transitional difficulty of adapting from home life to life at school, the actual process was made even more difficult by the distances most children had to travel for education. Even if the child was not at boarding school, a substantial journey to and from school was usually involved. This made a school day more tiring, and also had an effect on the child's opportunity for developing friendships and a social network. Making friends on a short walk to school is a natural experience for hearing children, but even this was difficult for the deaf children. Thus the natural stages of increased socialisation and play were either not established easily or artificially created by the educational opportunities available at the time.

Adolescence

The Chambers Twentieth Century Dictionary (1983) definition of adolescence is, 'passing from childhood to maturity'. It can be described as a phase of intensive physical and social change which may place great demands upon the individual and present many challenges. The child reaches puberty and with that comes the maturation of primary and secondary sex characteristics. Generally for girls this occurs between the ages of 10 to 15 years, while for boys the age range is 12 to 16 years.

Of interest to us is the relationship between the physical changes and the psychological changes and how these might impinge upon the response to remediation in communication impairment. Because of substantial changes to the physique the adolescent may become extremely self-conscious about the differences and this may result in worry and anxiety. Comparing self to others is common and this may increase self-consciousness if the adolescent perceives there to be great difference. For example, those who are atypically tall, short or overweight may suffer great distress. If the adolescent is further burdened by differences that are the result of disability, the suffering may be even greater if the individual has insight. People with stuttering problems, for example, are having to cope with an embarrassing difficulty with communication at a time when they are already extremely self-conscious about their self-presentation. As Schwartz (1993) states, the adolescent with a stuttering difficulty has to deal with and adjust to the speech difficulty, changing emotions and the relationship between the two. Various authors have argued that adolescents who have stuttering difficulties form a special group because of their vulnerable stage in life transition. This relates not only to the condition of stuttering itself, but also to the individual's response to any sort of remediation offered. Is the adolescent so self-conscious and anxious that attempts to remediate exacerbate the difficulty rather than facilitate improvement? In addition, as Schwartz points out, transfer and maintenance strategies may be threatened by adolescence. The younger adolescent may be able to accept reminders and instructions from parents, for example, but older adolescents do not want to be constantly reminded about their fluency levels, particularly from parents. Schwartz does recommend that peers can often be more helpful here. The adolescent wants to be part of a group and wants to identify with the peer group. At the same time the adolescent stutterer feels set apart from friends because of perceiving him or herself as different. In order to enable identification with peers, Schwartz suggests that bringing a friend to therapy sessions may be beneficial, as this then makes the stuttering problem more open and more shared. Transfer and maintenance can then take place more successfully.

Recent psychological research has focused on the experience of adolescence and its social implications. Jackson and Rodriguez-Tome (1993) discuss the social implications of reaching the period of adolescence. At this stage life becomes much more complex; relationships with parents change as the individual moves towards greater independence and peers occupy a much more central role in the individual's life. More time is spent with friends or alone and the amount of time spent with parents diminishes. The adolescent responds to external demands in school settings, and becomes more and more aware of the wider environment and its possibilities and limitations. All of the expansion and change of social worlds have implications for the experience of the communicatively impaired individual.

Worthington (1989) reports on the special difficulties experienced by adolescents in their recovery from traumatic brain injury. Adolescence has already been described in terms of the emotional turmoil associated with the physical changes. Adapting to a new body image may become an insurmountable difficulty if the adolescent becomes disabled. The problems in adapting to the new image can result in a poor self-image, self-consciousness and feelings of insecurity. In a discussion on two cases of adolescents suffering a severe head injury, Worthington describes the difficulties both subjects experienced. These related particularly to the disability and its capacity to take away almost all of the life experiences of normal adolescence. For example, both cases had to live with their families in a physically dependent situation. Both needed help with the most basic bodily functions and lost all hope of financial and living independence. Sexual development and expression was limited and the chances of a mature relationship in the future were very limited indeed. The conclusion that Worthington reached was that recovery from traumatic head injury was critically difficult in the more mature person, but with the adolescent, who is in a period of physical and emotional change, adaptation to circumstances is even more difficult to resolve. The normal maturational stages in adolescence cannot follow a successful progress and maladaptation may result.

Acquiring and losing

One of the main themes which runs through life relates to the notion of acquisition of skills (as in childhood development) and roles and status, and loss (as in loss of all of those things usually in later life). These are difficult concepts to deal with. Loss is usually associated with negativity. If you lose a role in life, such as a job, this is generally perceived as a difficult and negative time. Acquiring skills or material possessions which help to enhance identity is something which is usually much easier to deal with. However, it is argued that this is an entrenched way of viewing things. Losing a role may not necessarily be negative. It is partly cultural and sociological beliefs that cause people to believe this and many therapeutic interventions in counselling have to be directed towards enabling the individual to view a loss as a positive outcome which helps development, rather than as negative.

Loss and grief as a state of transition

Generally we view grief as something we experience when a loved one dies. Yet we can grieve for other things too. Some people may grieve for the loss of a loved pet. Others will grieve for the loss of a job. Grief occurs in many health care situations. Speck (1978) wrote extensively about the occurrence of loss within the medical setting. The field of obstetrics and gynaecology has a large literature on recognising and dealing with grief in relationship to the loss of a baby, whether as a miscarriage, at full-term or by abortion, and loss associated with hysterectomy. Other surgical procedures in medical contexts also generate grief, from surgery which removes a functional ability such as when a colostomy is carried out, to surgery which affects the individual's self-presentation as in face or neck surgery.

A similar parallel has been drawn in stroke, where the individual experiences loss of abilities such as mobility and independence. Here the individual has to cope with rehabilitation procedures while a carrying a memory of how life was before the stroke. Feelings of frustration, anger and depression are commonly associated with stroke and it is increasingly recognised that stroke patients need specific emotional support. In many studies following the descriptive work by Speck, the recognition and treatment of the emotional and social consequences of stroke is demonstrated to be critically important.

Murray Parkes (1975) has written about the process of grief in relation to work with the widowed and work with amputees. Seven components of grief are defined.

1   A process of realisation, i.e. the way in which the bereaved moves from denial or avoidance of recognition of the loss towards acceptance.
2   An alarm reaction – anxiety, restlessness, and the physiological accompaniments of fear.
3   An urge to search for and to find the lost person in some form.
4   Anger and guilt, including outbursts directed against those who press the bereaved person towards premature acceptance of his loss.
5   Feelings of internal loss of self or guilt.
6   Identification phenomena – the adoption of traits, mannerisms or symptoms of the lost person, with or without a sense of his or her presence within the self.
7   Pathological variants of grief, i.e. the reaction may be excessive and prolonged or inhibited and inclined to emerge in a distorted form.

Clearly, losing a leg is not exactly the same as losing a spouse. As Murray Parkes says, 'I don't love my left leg, at least not in the same way as I love my wife' (p. 213). Yet Murray Parkes outlines the various experiences of the amputees and compares them with the experiences of the widows, and there is a striking similarity. Looking initially at the first component, both groups were reported as going through a process of realisation, where coming to understand the actuality of the loss varies between individuals. Murray Parkes reports that 39 per cent of the 56 amputees reported a feeling of numbness, all of the group had a feeling of the persisting presence of the lost limb, and 87 per cent reported how they often forgot that the limb was missing and went to use it. Although this relates to the phenomenon of the phantom limb, Murray Parkes argues that this is influenced by psychological factors. Other similarities with the remaining components are also discussed.

Worden (1982) describes the components of grief as consisting of four major categories: 1) feelings, 2) physical sensations, 3) cognitions, and 4) behaviours. This very detailed analysis of the experience of grief gives useful explanations about the complex way in which people experience loss. Worden describes the most commonly reported physical sensations experienced as part of grieving (p. 24):

•   hollowness in the stomach
•   tightness in the chest

- tightness in the throat
- over-sensitivity to noise
- a sense of depersonalisation: 'I walk down the street and nothing seems real, including myself'
- breathlessness, feeling short of breath
- weakness in the muscles
- lack of energy
- dry mouth.

As Worden notes, these symptoms may be perceived by individuals to be health concerns and frequently they will ask the doctor for help for the physical symptom. Many newly bereaved people also report that their thoughts are confused. Loss of concentration is a commonly reported problem, as in what Worden describes as 'preoccupation' – obsession with thoughts about the deceased. Hallucinations are also included and these refer to both the visual type and the auditory type, occurring within a few weeks following the loss. Depressive thought patterns are also common, where the bereaved will find thoughts recurring such as, 'I can't live without her' or 'I'll never find love again'.

Tanner and Gerstenberger (1988) wrote a controversial paper outlining the dimensions of loss experienced by the person who becomes communicatively handicapped by a stroke. Three aspects to the loss are reported: that of person, self and object. Loss of person refers to psychological separation from loved ones which occurs because of the communicative impairment. It is impossible to maintain the same equality of relationship because direct communication becomes so difficult. Loss of self occurs when the individual recognises that aspects of physical and psychological integrity are no longer there. Tanner and Gerstenberger report that the point at which the individual recognises he or she does not have the functional capabilities of others is the critical point when grief for loss of self is most intensely felt. Loss of object refers to a loss such as enjoyment of sophisticated use of the computer which becomes impossible if the individual has acquired language problems. Thus a valued object and experience is lost and severely affects the quality of the individual's life.

As can be seen, grief is a multifaceted emotion; it encompasses a whole series of feelings which can occur in phases or overlap. Tanner and Gerstenberger interpret grief in the following stages.

Denial

This is usually the first stage in the reaction. Here the individual denies the existence of the condition, as in the following example:

> I do not have a speech-language disorder. The problems occurring with communication are a result of the listener's inability or unwillingness to understand my perfectly normal communicative attempts. (p. 81)

Second, the individual perceives the speech-language impairment as a temporary and insignificant problem which will go away spontaneously. This is described as partial denial. Another way of denying is by believing that external factors will clear up the problem, such as the belief that an external god will make things right again. Here the individual is aware that the communication problem exists but that 'supernatural' forces will overcome the problem and so relieve the individual of any need to work at recovery.

Finally, denial may be seen in the individual who has the following sort of belief:

> I have a significant speech and language disorder, but through my determination I will overcome it and be just like I was before the brain damage. (p. 82)

According to Tanner and Gerstenberger, this theme of denial is employed by individuals whose pre-morbid locus of control was internal. The denial aspect rests in the fact that if the individual believes that commitment of personal work on recovery will solve the problems, then this leaves no psychological room for spontaneous recovery or more seriously, no recovery.

Denial in any of these ways can be viewed as a buffer to psychological pain. It permits the individual time to develop psychological adaptation to the condition and as such should be viewed as an often necessary process. Tanner and Gerstenberger warn against the difference between misinformation and denial in the responses of patients to the condition. That is, if the patient has been misinformed about the course of recovery their reactions will be based on the misinformation, whereas in denial the information may be correct but it is the patient's interpretation which is the issue.

Frustration

This is described as occurring in two ways. First, frustration about being unable to communicate as once was possible; second, frustration about being unable to change the course of events which have led to the losses. Every time the patient is confronted with a reminder of the loss, such as trying to answer the telephone, frustration occurs because there is no way of altering events to make this difficulty go away. Anger is a typical reaction to frustration.

Depression

Awareness of a major loss frequently leads to depression. This may be short lived or longer and more difficult for both the aphasic speaker and carers to deal with. The depression can create cognitive, physical and emotional reactions, and is linked to the process of realisation which the patient moves through as a way of understanding the loss. What is difficult in this is that some patients may move successfully through the process of realisation and gradually move out of depression, whereas others may be unable to leave the depressive state. In a normal grieving process depression can be seen to be normal and a productive experience because it gives the individual time to come to terms with what has happened. Thus, in normal circumstances, as Tanner and Gerstenberger say, 'Depression is the natural reaction to conscious awareness of significant loss' (p. 83).

Acceptance

If the patient is able to move successfully through all stages of the grieving process, acceptance should occur. Tanner and Gerstenberger emphasise the difference between acceptance and resignation, where acceptance is a positive state, a 'goal of grieving' (p. 83). Resignation has a more negative value; it represents having to put up with something. Tanner and Gerstenberger acknowledge that acceptance may not always be achieved but that it needs to be a goal for all patients.

Brumfitt and Clarke (1983) also outlined the meaning of loss in the context of the aphasic's experience, and identified specific losses. These were:

- loss of capacity for everyday and essential communication, e.g. asking ward staff for a drink
- asking questions to medical staff about the condition, being assertive and requesting information, as normally happens when the patient is a normal speaker
- the loss of quality in personal relationships in the sense that joining in exchange of loving affectionate conversation with relatives, e.g. the relative can say 'take care' at the end of visiting while in hospital but the aphasic speaker may be unable to return this
- reading the words on get-well cards, receiving and making telephone calls
- expressing anger – we usually rely on verbal means to disclose our anger. People with aphasic problems may have to resort to non-verbal means to express anger and may be misperceived because of it. Others may interpret them as childish or regressed and thus the aphasic speaker may be managed and interacted with in a different way to those with intact linguistic skills
- teasing and joking – this is an important part of human relationships which may be inaccessible to aphasic speakers, as it may require too high a level of fluency.

Grieving, of course, is not the exclusive preserve of aphasic speakers. Many people with communication problems grieve either for what they once had or for what they might have been had they not been handicapped by communication disorder. People who experience laryngectomy operations will feel the loss of the normal capacity to communicate and as Dalton (1994) reports, it is a loss which cannot be restored. Other forms of dysphonia refer to more temporary problems which, with intervention, can facilitate the return of normal voice. However, the loss of voice, even temporary, can affect the individual's self-perception and create a difficult point in their movement through life.

People who have stuttering difficulties may have known no other way of communicating, but even so may have to deal with complex feelings of loss about what might have been had they been fluent speakers. Many people with stuttering difficulties work in contexts which have been chosen to avoid confrontational speaking situations. Thus the person with a stuttering problem who works in a computing situation may have real leanings towards being a school teacher, but does not choose to become one because of the stuttering. If the individual finds this difficult to accept, in spite of it being a realistic decision, then the feelings of loss may never be resolved without help.

Carers of people with communication problems

Spouses and carers of aphasic speakers and others with acquired disorders are frequently observed to go through a parallel grief reaction. The spouse will experience loss of the person who was there before the stroke and at the same time the loss of the relationship. Anderson (1992) discusses the loss of quality of life experienced by carers of stroke patients. In a major study of 176 patients with stroke, the results demonstrated that life changed substantially and detrimentally for the carer regardless of degree of the patient's disability. Shontz (1965) described four stages that family members experience as a reaction to the sudden impairment in communication of one member: shock, realisation, retreat and acknowledgement. As Rollin (1987) states, the carers may get stuck at any point along these stages and be unable to move on and cope without professional help. Kinsella and Duffy (1979) found psychiatric disorders in wives of aphasic speakers which related to the increased demands placed upon them, the social isolation and increasing guilt and resentment about the situation they were now placed in.

The parents of a child who is born with some handicap may experience feelings of loss about the perfect child they had longed for. Loss of the ideal child is often referred to in literature. Here the parents have to come to terms with the nature of the handicap the child has which may involve a long protracted diagnosis even before a clear understanding of the child's problem can be found. Thus juggling strong feelings about a child who may be permanently handicapped has to be dealt with while the parent deals with grief over how they imagined their child was going to be. It is not suggested that this grief is a conscious experience unless help is provided. This may relate only to submerged feelings but they may have a power to influence the way the parent copes. Rollin (1987, p. 246) discusses the grieving mother who is so much caught up in guilt, sorrow, mourning, anger and apprehension that a 'warm nurturing relationship' may be disrupted or never be achieved successfully.

Other work referred to by Rollin outlines the ways in which parents move through the stages in coming to terms with their child's handicap. The success of moving through these stages is dependent on several inter-related factors, including:

1   the mental health of individual family members
2   the nature of the marital relationship
3   the ability to cope with stress
4   the quality and degree of deformity
5   the nature of and degree to which the family receives information about the deformity and possible sequelae
6   the effectiveness of the rehabilitation team. (p. 233)

Clearly all professionals have to be aware of these factors in order to be most effective with parents. Dalton (1994) also refers to the parents' unresolved grief that needs to be addressed in order to let them eventually come to terms with their child's handicap. Frequently parents feel responsible for the handicap although there is no logical way in which they actually have responsibility. For example, a child born with a genetic condition may leave the parents feeling guilt ridden and responsible for the damaged life of their child, although clearly they are not in fact guilty of causing the handicap to be there. Dalton reports that this situation can often be seen in a mother who is so guilt ridden that she refuses to allow anyone to look after her disabled child. By enabling the mother to experiment with leaving her child to the care of others and obtaining respite care, Dalton suggests that she will be able to resolve the grief and embedded guilt and cope more productively herself, while giving her child a better opportunity for independent development.

Ageing in the context of life transitions

It has been suggested that the study of the psychology of ageing is best placed within the study of the whole life span. Instead of adults who suddenly change categories and become 'old people', a more coherent view is of the older person moving into this last phase as a natural part of development.

This last phase of 'integrity' is a highly complex phase. The older person is required to achieve successful integrity within the context of all the physical, cognitive and social changes that take place as part of normal 'ageing'. It may also need to be achieved while health deterio-rates.

It is assumed that the older person experiences inner changes associated with the different goals in life, such as how to spend retirement, where to live and so on. These inner changes may be successful if the person is able to reflect on and confront aspects of their past life, without shame, regret or guilt. But the older person who cannot confront the past life, or is distressed because of it, may be unable to achieve 'integrity' and experience only 'despair' (Erikson 1980). As Coleman (1993, p. 87) states, there is no guarantee either, that society is organised so as to encourage older people to develop the qualities necessary for integrity:

> Successful ageing depends on the satisfactory resolution of issues raised earlier in life, but this internal development is itself dependent on the opportunities and encouragement provided in the person's present environment.

Coleman also refers to a study which used observers' reports of personality over a longitudinal study of 50 years. Older people were rated significantly more open minded, cheerful and accepting, which was interpreted in terms of Erikson's theory of 'integrity' in the last phase of life.

Integrity versus despair, according to Erikson, centres around the individual's capacity to accept and make sense of their life, now that it has reached the final stage. Salmon (1985) discusses a case described by Oliver Sachs (1976) in the remarkable discussion of patients who were 'awakened' after receiving the miracle drug L-DOPA. One lady who had developed Parkinson's disease type symptoms had become more and more incapacitated, ending up immobile, speechless and unreachable. Her admission to hospital was followed by the complete break-up of her family. When she was given L-DOPA in old age, she became completely different. As well as suffering extreme emotions and hallucinations, and bizarre involuntary movements, she experienced good periods of equilibrium where she came gradually to understand her situation. Salmon comments on how, over time, she was able to accept things as they were and achieve a personal stability.

Here is a remarkable event which is notable for its association with the theoretical description of transitional stages. Even in such extreme circumstances, this lady was able successfully to move towards psychologically healthy old age.

Clearly, ageing is not just about increasing the number of years one is alive. Ageing is a multifaceted event involving physical, cognitive, behavioural and psychosocial changes. The ways in which the individual is affected are purely idiosyncratic and influenced by many external factors such as socioeconomic status, inherited factors, physical conditions, health status and life experiences. Normal changes, like these described, may be accompanied by pathological problems such as heart disease, stroke, cancer, changes in immunity, arthritis and changes to sensory abilities such as loss of hearing and vision.

For the reader who is learning about the health care context, the expectations about reaching old age need to be considered in the light of this multifactorial status of ageing. Growing old can be explained in descriptive terms, but the meaning of being old has to be understood within an understanding of what being old means to that individual. Finding out the personal meaning of ageing may be simple with some patients in a health care setting. With some, it can be introduced into the conversation easily. For the communicatively handicapped individual though, this is much more difficult. Being old may mean you have to cope with differing cognitive changes which may occur as the result of illness, such as stroke and associated communication problems, Alzheimer's disease and other degenerative conditions.

The child with language impairment: growing older

There is some indication that a child with a communication impairment may have associated behavioural or emotional problems. Coping with a complicated communication impairment must clearly have effects upon the interpersonal life of the child and moving through the different transitional stages must be more difficult than for a child with normal abilities. Professionally, we do not, however, refer to the child with communication impairment in the context of the life transitions. Although a useful structure, the speech and language therapy context rarely uses this for increasing professional insight.

There are some indications that a child with a communication impairment may develop behavioural problems which increase with age. Although this area is underdeveloped, Stevenson, Richman and Grahame (1985) reported a study which looked at the association between behaviour problems and language abilities at three years and behavioural difficulties at eight years. A sample of 535 children were followed from their third birthday to their eighth birthday. At age three, mothers were interviewed at home and data was collected on the child's reported behaviour development and family background. Three measures of language development were used which captured the ability to show understanding of single words, naming ability and structural ability demonstrated by results from the Reynell development language scales (Reynell 1969). The authors stressed that this was merely a screening procedure and could not distinguish severity or type of language impairment. At age eight, data was collected by using the Rutter teacher's scale (Rutter 1967), a questionnaire designed to identify children with behavioural deviance.

The results showed that behaviour problems at three would have predicted 56 per cent of the behaviour problems which were identified at eight years of age. It was of interest that language structure as assessed on the screening assessment was more closely related to the behavioural deviance. It is suggested that language structure is more closely related to the ability of the child to formulate ideas and thoughts and this has a bearing on the child's capacity to make successful interpersonal relationships in the long term. Clearly this needs further investigation, but it is an interesting conclusion.

In addition, the authors discuss the emergence of behavioural difficulties in the context of transmission into school. It is suggested that expectations about behaviour on transferring to school at age five may mask true behavioural difficulties which only emerge after the family have assumed that the child's behaviour is related to learning to cope in school.

Summary

The individual may move smoothly or uncomfortably through the various stages of life. In addition, all of us have to face unpredictable challenges which may enforce transitional states that may be painful. To what extent all of these factors can influence a client's response to therapy and the therapist's response to the client has to be reflected on in the future. Some useful research could take these ideas forward and give us increased understanding into the world of the person with a communication impairment. How might the individual with a communication impairment experience a disrupted biography? Does having a communication impairment make it more difficult to reflect? We can predict that therapeutic intervention can provide help to ease the individual's pain and to help the individual confront the new challenges, but we still need to be able to prove this conclusively.

Exercises

When you became a student your life changed. List:

1 the good aspects to this
2 the bad aspects to this.

Looking back, was this a time of difficult transition for you or not?

Recommended reading

Cohen LH (1988) Life Events and Psychological Functioning. London: Sage.
Salmon P (1985) Living in Time. London: JM Dent and Sons.
Worden JW (1983) Grief Counselling and Grief Therapy. London: Tavistock Publications.

Chapter 4
The Family

Overview

This chapter will enable you to:

- gain a psychological understanding of factors which affect families
- understand what contributes to well-functioning families and families where there are problems
- understand the role of the family in relation to the client with a communication handicap and how the family may or may not facilitate improvement.

Introduction

The child you see in the clinic has significant signs of non-fluency with prolongations of sounds initially. He is the eldest of three brothers who are all under the age of seven and his parents are in their early 20s. His father has a mild stuttering difficulty that he reports was helped by speech and language therapy when he was a child. The father works as a long-distance lorry driver and is away from home for a lot of the week, returning usually at weekends. The mother is clearly stressed and rather angry.

The child with the fluency problem is shy with you and unhappy to speak. When he refuses to speak his mother becomes very irritated with him and tells him that he must. She says, 'If you don't speak I won't buy you any sweets when we leave here.'

This child may have an inherited predisposition to develop a stuttering problem. Is this the only issue when considering his difficulties? Does his family context have any concerns for you? What might you want to take into consideration here?

What is a family?

We can liken the family to a machine which relies on the action of all its parts for smooth functioning. (Altschuler 1997, p. 39)

We all have different experiences of being part of a family and can view it from many perspectives – from being a child growing up to being the parent and learning how to care for developing children. In different cultures there are different expectations of the family unit, particularly with reference to the closeness and responsibilities between generations. In this society we normally expect the family to include two parents and a number of children ranging from one to usually no more than five. Yet, given the high divorce rate and the increasing numbers of lone parents, the conventional family unit has recently been described as being unrepresentative of society as a whole. As there is an increase in lone parents, there is also an increase in children living as stepchildren in family units where one parent has formed a new relationship with another person who then becomes stepparent. All of these new forms of family unit can be strong and valid ways of bringing up children, but clearly the possibility of complications arising in these units is recognised and these will be discussed.

It is important to acknowledge that being part of a family (however that is configured) is a core part of the person's understanding of self. In reality most of the individual's survival and development depends upon the family unit. The most obvious way is for physical care but we also know that the way in which the individual develops an identity is based upon the experiences gained while growing up in a family. Recognising self in the context of the family is a way of defining the self-concept as psychological reality, as in 'Family self', the section devoted to this in the Tennessee self-concept scale (Roid and Fitts 1994) that refers to the perception of one's sense of adequacy, worth and value as a family member. This recognition of self within the family context and its role as a core of personal understanding demonstrates the importance of the family to all clients who we may come across in our professional life.

The primary relationship is seen as critical in the infant's early years. Usually this is with the mother, but there are many alternatives in primary relationships depending on the social circumstances of the infant. This is frequently referred to as the attachment phase and relates to the infant's first experience of care and love. Its function is described as providing a possible prototype for future relationships and an emotional context with stability for the growing infant. As the infant matures, more people become reliable and safe to be with and, if development is successful, the child will grow to feel secure with a variety of people.

Social learning is also a necessary part of development of the individual and much of this takes place within the family setting. Children are 'taught' to be civilised, codes of conduct are learnt; thus attitudes and values are all basic qualities which come from the individual's existence in a family unit. The child learns to adapt behaviour to the 'rules' set out by the family and relies on feedback from parents or care givers about what is acceptable and what is not. For the majority of families, there is an aversion to antisocial behaviour and for the majority the drive within the family is for the developing child to learn skills for appropriate behaviour within the social context.

Rollin (1987) discusses the health of the family in western society and refers to Fogarty (1976) who describes the ideal family and how it functions. This definition describes the family as adaptable and responsive to any change. For example, a child with special needs would have effects upon the family function and have cause to make the family respond to changes. The definition also refers to emotional problems which may exist in the family unit but need to be dealt with by the family and are altered by the way family members cope. In other words, if the family does not deal with the problems then it could no longer continue to exist in its present form. Individual differences are emphasised and recognised by a strong family unit. Each person is identified as different and allowed to develop in the way that he or she wishes. All of the health of a family depends on the enjoyment by each member of the family of each other, and of the family as a whole. Any one family member feels free to use any other family member for feedback and learning with no fear of embarrassment or criticism. Fogarty, who wrote this in the context of family therapy, also discussed the effects of a dispute between parents and the importance of ensuring the resolution should not involve any child being used to solve the problem.

Parenting

The art or skill of parenting has vexed generations of parents for hundreds of years. In the past it has almost seemed a haphazard chance that individuals should become good citizens following their upbringing. Nowadays more is known about the ways in which children respond to styles of parenting, but even so the influence of the behaviours of parents is still not sufficiently disentangled. For example, children may grow into adults who mirror their parents' views. Yet other children may grow into adults determined to represent the opposite of their parents' views. If two people with differing experiences of being parented marry, then we are uncertain how these different styles may be resolved for the new generation of children. Inconsistent handling by parents is frequently a causative factor in behavioural problems and family distress.

Duck (1986) and Smith, Cowie and Blades (1998) discuss three key styles of parenting which have been defined. These are based on work by Baumrind (1973) who, by means of interviews and observations, obtained data about child-rearing practices of the mothers and fathers of 134 preschool children, focusing on four dimensions of parenting behaviour. These were control, nurturance, clarity of communication and maturity demands. First, there are authoritarian parents who try to control and evaluate the behaviour of their children, stressing obedience to a set of their chosen parental standards. Punishment takes the form of physical or psychological methods (such as withdrawal of love). Second, permissive parents are very accepting of their children's behaviour and believe in reasoning with the child as a way of motivating them. The third approach relates to being authoritative rather than authoritarian and aims to direct the children through a process of reasoning and firm control. Duck points out that this differs in style from permissiveness in that the relationship is not based upon equality but by verbal control without psychological manipulation. The children brought up by this method of parenting are more likely to be independent, cooperative and friendly.

Apart from the importance of defining the parental styles, the research points to characteristics that can be expected in children when brought up by one of these styles. The children of authoritarian parents tend to have children who are difficult, dependent and socially incompetent. Children brought up by permissive parents are most likely to be generally unmotivated, not interested or enthusiastic about achievement. Children of authoritative parents have been found to be the most competent; they tend to be more self-reliant, keen to achieve, co-operative with both adults and children and socially responsible. Clearly the implications of parenting styles upon the outcome of therapy is critical, but in a clinical setting we have to be cautious about how we find out this information. Parents do not, on the whole, have enough self-awareness to understand what style of parenting they are using. It may be automatic and dependent upon what they experienced as a child. Thus, clinically, observation and careful questioning may lead to insight for the therapist and eventually to increased insight for the parent.

Are there any differences between the way a mother relates to a child and the way a father does?

Studies (Lewis 1986) have shown that fathers tend to interact with their young children in a more physical way; that is with rough and tumble activities such as chasing, bouncing and tossing the child in the air. Mothers are observed to be more gentle and more verbal, using toys and verbal interaction to relate to the child. Frequently, this has been debated in terms of whether this is learned behaviour by parents who have observed their own parents behaving like this, or whether this is owing to sex difference. According to Schaffer (1996) there is little support for this latter argument when physiological measurements are taken as a way of showing differences in responsiveness to pictures of babies who have a variety of facial expressions such as crying or smiling. If physiological arousal patterns of heart rate and blood pressure are used as indicators then no significant differences are shown between the sexes.

But we have society which is changing in terms of the way we take care of our children. Are fathers who stay at home to look after their children likely to develop different ways of behaving towards young children because of this? How many speech and language therapists now interview the father as the main care taker when working in the paediatric setting?

Field (1978) explored the behaviour of fathers who were the primary caretakers and compared them with fathers who were secondary and mothers who were primary. The conclusions reached were that fathers who were primary caretakers showed similar behaviours to the mothers who were primary, and therefore behaved differently from the fathers who were secondary.

When one of the parents is a stepparent, then the family relationships may change. Various studies have been completed to look at the effects upon children in this type of family unit. As Smith et al. (1998) report, some of the evidence is conflicting. Luepnitz (1986) showed some very positive aspects of the new living arrangements for children who were compared in groups of those who were in sole custody with the mother, sole custody with the father and in joint custody, two years or more after the separation. Measures of child adjustment were found to be independent of custody type. Joint custody had the advantage of the child developing independent relationships with both natural parents, and also reduced many financial and parenting pressures. But there are obvious advantages to single custody should the wife need protecting from possible abuse.

Problems in families

All families have problems and cope with the difficulties within the unit, or at least with temporary external support or advice. However, families can break down for a variety of reasons and these need to be addressed in the context of understanding what influences these situations may have on the client with communication handicap.

Abuse of children

Society today has begun to confront the problem of child abuse in a way previously unheard of. Social history has recorded maltreatment of children from many times and cultures where this was commonplace and uncontroversial. What seems to be striking in the reports referred to in many textbooks is how slowly public opinion moved towards a realisation that this was unacceptable. Some of the descriptions seem outrageous now. Gillham (1994) reported on the legal status of a child. Until 1824 it was not an offence, under English Law, to steal a child (no value) unless he or she were clothed. If the child was clothed the person taking the child could be convicted of stealing the clothes. In the late 1800s legislation was brought in to protect the child and many convictions for deliberate cruelty were brought even in the late 1800s. However, as Gillham notes, although deliberate cruelty to children was recognised, neglect was still unexplored in this country. In order to recognise this, the government passed the Children's Act in 1908 which sought to give children social rights independent of their parents. This proved to be a turning point in our attitudes to children but, even so, confronting the issues around deliberate physical abuse by parents towards children and sexual abuse has still emerged relatively slowly.

Physical abuse

Suspected cases of child abuse and neglect are required to be referred to social services departments and have to be investigated. Usually a case conference considers evidence and decides what action should be taken, for example, placing the child and family name on the child protection register. Physical abuse is generally classified within a number of groups which include sexual abuse, neglect (this refers to health and safety problems, such as accidental injury, care and nutrition), emotional abuse (mental cruelty but acknowledged to be difficult to define), grave concern (previously the at-risk register) and general physical abuse.

The Department of Health keeps records of children registered from all social work departments in England, but not Wales or Scotland (see Figure 4.1). These are published in the form of annual reports, but the information in these is limited. Gillham (1994) records that there is little information about the nature of the abuse apart from the category of registration and the parental and social circumstances of the children. There is little research which provides information about the true incidence and prevalence of abuse in children, although clearly there is a lot more interest now than even ten years ago. One of the methodological problems is the difficulty in the detectibility of abuse. It may not be identified as abuse, or even if it is identified, it is not necessarily reported to child protection agencies and not all of those reported are registered.

Sex
Boys   16,400
Girls   15,700

Category of abuse
Neglect   12,200
Physical   10,900
Sexual   7,400
Emotional   5,000
Grave concern   –
Other   600

Figure 4.1. Children and young people on child protection registers at 31 March 1997 (figures represent 29 children in every 10,000).
Source: Health and Personal Social Services Statistics for England 1997.

Non-accidental injury

Recognition of abuse to children is the responsibility of all members of the public, but clearly observations of this may occur in professional contexts such as therapy. The actual responsibility for diagnosis of non-accidental injury lies with the medical profession and expertise and technology (for example, skilled interpretation of X-ray material) is critical. Unfortunately, the diagnosis still remains one of medical *interpretation* rather than absolute scientific proof. The initial steps towards diagnosis are strongly influenced by the history obtained from the parents. Because of the sensitive nature of the interview, many parents are reluctant to provide information or may create reasons for the injury which may be unlikely. Bamford (1989) notes that even if the history obtained is factually inaccurate, the manner in which it is given is particularly important. For example, some parents may be full of remorse and open about the situation whereas others may try to deny the incident or even display disinterest by sending other offspring to the hospital instead of attending themselves. Clearly interviewing parents about potential non-accidental injury is not the role of the speech and language therapist; however, it is important to be aware of the procedures involved. Non-accidental injury relates to injuries in the following categories.

- head injuries produced by direct trauma or acceleration or deceleration of the head
- bone injuries including multiple fractures which are more extensive than would have been expected from the type of injury reported
- soft tissue injuries such as bruising, scratches and injury to the mouth
- burns
- injuries of the abdomen and chest, which are more unusual, but may be the result of blows and may require urgent life saving treatment.

Child/infant mortality

The issue within this category focuses on whether death occurs as a result of a critical moment of physical abuse or as the result of neglect which may take place over time. Another factor of concern as reported by Gillham (1994) is that a substantial number of child mortalities which occur as a result of abuse are from families not known to any child protection agency or register. The majority of children who die as the result of abuse are young, usually under two or three years old, and many studies record boys as being in the majority.

Divorce and family breakdown

Because of the increasing numbers of divorces, research has been done to identify predictors and factors which may contribute to a marital breakdown. It is known that the poor and the poorly educated and those who marry young are more likely to have higher divorce rates than better educated people. Also, the marital success or failure of a couple's own parents affects the chance of breakdown. The factors which indicate a strong relationship are the capacity to communicate well, providing each other with emotional support and coping in a constructive way with conflict and challenging situations. The implications of this for the marriage when one of the partners loses the ability to cope for medical reasons, such as following stroke, must be acknowledged. When one partner suffers a stroke the aftermath may be extremely difficult to deal with. The unaffected partner has to take responsibility for all aspects of their everyday life as well as providing emotional and physical support. How the couple have previously handled difficulty may influence how well they cope with the major changes following the stroke. If successful marriages rely on good communication between the partners then communication difficulties caused by brain damage will certainly exacerbate other problems.

In terms of the progress of events associated with couples becoming divorced from each other, Bohannon (1971) refers to six processes that have to be moved through in order to deal with the predicament. These are:

- the emotional divorce which relates to the conflict, ending of communication and antagonism towards each other
- the legal divorce which may have emotional implications for individuals as well as legal realities
- the economic divorce which may create tensions between the two parties and therefore cause further emotional distress
- the coparental divorce which deals with the custody issues of the children and produces great emotional strain
- the community divorce which relates to the individual status within the community and the necessary adaptations to this
- the psychic divorce which involves the issue of regaining personal autonomy.

Clearly, the problems for the children within this situation can be huge. If the children perceived their family situation to be safe and happy then they may be extremely unsettled by the divorce and the loss of the security they believed in. Duck (1986) reports that children of divorcing parents experience depression and psychological disturbance including guilt that the divorce may be their fault. Some children may be expected to 'take sides' by their parents, or even be on the receiving end of displaced aggression from their parents. The status of children within their social context is threatened as well as in their actual family situation, and thus the loss of the family as it once was may cause immense emotional changes for children. Children may perceive themselves as coming from a 'broken home' or being the 'children of divorced parents'. These labels are painful statements about the child's new status and are difficult to shake off. If the parents remarry then the children also have to adjust to new relationships and this may also be a critical time for them.

Dysfunctional families

Duck (1986) describes the features of families in which the functioning is wrong and may cause problems in the future for their members. If the family focuses on the negative aspects of a situation then this will contribute to problems. Parents who are poor observers of their children's behaviour may not be able to identify changes and therefore provide poor feedback to the developing child (this relates specifically to understanding the context of the child with communication difficulties; think of the example at the beginning of this chapter). If the parents are inconsistent in the way they deal with misbehaviour, the children in the family will not learn the rules and so grow up confused. Children need positive affection and praise and things may be problematic if these are not forthcoming from parents. Also if the emphasis is on power between the parents and children (i.e. 'Don't think you can say you can go on that day trip because it is expensive and I am the one with the money') the relationships will be poor.

Not all dysfunctional family problems result from parental mismanagement. Disruptive children cause reactions in their parents that in turn reflect back upon the child. Children with specific problems that may be congenital can affect the family functioning regardless of the level of skill of the parents.

The gifted child

As well as recognising the predicament of the child who suffers environmental difficulties such as exposure to violence in the family, there are other children who are special because of their gifts. Although it is hard to show predictive factors which influence the occurrence of gifted children, Radford (1990) stated that there are two ways in which families can influence excellence in their children: first, by specific teaching of skills and knowledge, and second by transmitting values and attitudes about the importance of learning and so on. One study at the University of Chicago showed that although there were many differences between families of gifted children, there were similarities. All of the parents were very motivated for their children to succeed, whatever the background of the particular ability. For example, much time would be devoted to 'skilling' the child in the area in which he or she showed aptitude, for example music. The family would provide specialist teaching, arrange many extra curricular activities and provide praise. Time spent on the particular activity would be rewarded in some way. Although this pattern has emerged

there are few explanations (other than sociological) for why there so few
recorded gifted children from ethnic minorities and fewer girls than boys.

The family affected by chronic illness

Altschuler (1997) discusses the effects upon a family when one of its
members experiences chronic illness. Initially, the main consideration is
whether the condition is sudden (as in stroke) or consists of a slow build
up of symptoms (as in cases of cancer). In the case of a condition such as
stroke the family has to make huge adjustments in the early stages which
may then settle down as the symptoms stabilise. In the case of cancer the
family has to continually readjust and cope with new symptoms, a new
prognosis and prepare themselves, in some cases, for the death of the
family member. All of these factors will affect the organisation of the family,
both in terms of practical arrangements (i.e. who drives the car, takes the
children to school and so on) and in terms of the psychological roles that
people have (i.e. who has the responsibility for nurturing and comforting
people within the family). Ways of coping will vary from family to family,
but some will become more intimate as a strategy for coping with the
illness whereas others will show avoidance behaviour in either helping or
referring to the patient's condition.

Whether the symptoms are episodic or constant also affects the
functioning of the family in that members can lead their 'normal' lives
some of the time and then lead a life more specifically focused on the
family member when necessary. Illness such as kidney disease may have
special effects on family life as the whole family may have to organise
itself around the treatment regime of the patient. The amount of
incapacitation and symptom visibility will influence how the family
copes. If the patient is disabled, there are many issues to do with how
the family members feel about going out into society with the patient.
Children, for example, can often find this difficult if they feel embarrassed by the way the patient – their parent – looks. Altschuler quotes an
example of children who were acutely embarrassed by their mother who
had multiple sclerosis and was very clumsy in public. The mother is
reported as being more distressed by this than by the terminal quality of
her illness.

If the condition is a progressive one then the family has to move
towards coping with the eventual death of the family member. Here it is
particularly noticeable that the boundaries of the family become more
open and permeable. Doctors, nurses and other health care workers
become closely involved with the family and take on roles within that
structure. Issues which were previously discussed only with the family
are now discussed freely with these professionals. If the spouse is dying,
the other spouse may be unable to provide comfort to sustain the rest of
the family, and a professional may have to take on the role.

The family context for the aphasic speaker

Numerous discussions exist that explore the reactions of the family to aphasia in one of its members (Rollin 1987; Wahrborg 1991; Boisclair-Papillon 1993; Parr et al. 1997). All of these discussions refer to the major changes within the family unit which are mainly attributed to the onset of aphasia. Rollin (1987) reviews the most commonly reported early work on family reactions and refers to Malone (1969) where irritability, guilt, health problems, rejection and over solicitousness are frequently noted in the responses of relatives. Kinsella and Duffy (1979) report the feelings of isolation, anxiety and irritability as well as behaviours associated with overprotection and disordered interpersonal relationships. Shontz (1965) described the emotional process family members go through as shock, realisation, retreat and acknowledgement. In effect these are like the grief reactions of the individual aphasic speakers. The family can be seen to experience the same sort of feelings about the onset of aphasia and loss of the opportunity to communicate well.

Many of these reports of families do not represent empirical work but are qualitative reports from interviews. Boisclair-Papillon (1993) discusses the changes without data and refers to the loss of role frequently reported in studies. When individuals become aphasic their partners may have to take on roles that were previously those of the aphasic speaker. This particularly refers to roles which involve communicative ability, for example, financial aspects of a person's life, like organising personal bank accounts. Sometimes taking a new role may be fraught with difficulty in spite of the willingness of the unaffected partner to do this. Not all partners know the detail, for example, of their financial affairs. It is not unknown for partners to be unused to writing cheques, uncertain of how the insurance is paid, or even about details of the family business which are only known to the aphasic speaker. If the affected partner had suffered two broken legs it would be possible for the unaffected partner to pick up the reins with the verbal guidance from the patient. This may be impossible if the patient is communicatively handicapped. However, as Boisclair-Papillon notes, roles within family life are much more flexible now than in the past and many tasks are more easily taken on now than before. Boisclair-Papillon also refers to other difficulties, including the guilt experienced by many families alongside the tendency to overprotect the aphasic partner. Also, unrealistic attitudes may exist about the recovery potential of the aphasic person which may cause adjustment difficulties.

Personal intimacy is also lost as well as reported loss of sexual satisfaction. Kinsella and Duffy (1979) reported 83 per cent of the couples in their survey had abandoned sexual activity following the stroke. Wiig (1973) discusses the effects upon sexuality and notes that misunderstandings can occur as the result of diminished non-verbal ability; also hemiplegia in men can affect erectal function. Some reports refer to fear of orgasm following stroke because the mental experience feels similar. Social activities too are reported as decreasing, with an increasing sense of isolation.

Parr et al. (1997) state that stroke affects partnerships in the family in four main ways: communication, physical changes, emotional changes and role changes. If there are significant communication problems then the handicapped person may be unable to express everyday needs and personal feelings. The communication changes clearly affect the partner's relationship in the early days of coping, but as Parr et al. note, facing other challenging situations within the family can cause huge stresses, particularly if the aphasic speaker has insufficient language to express views. They quote a number of instances, such as when the aphasic person's partner becomes seriously ill and the aphasic person is unable to question the GP or understand explanations about what is happening. A particular situation is referred to where an aphasic woman was widowed after her husband had died of cancer. She had only been aphasic for a short while and found great difficulty in coping. Her difficulties in coping with loss of language (apart from the immense personal loss of her husband) were exacerbated by being without a partner to facilitate her speaking in social situations. Trying to rebuild her life after the loss of her husband was made exceptionally problematic because she had no communicative skills to help her make new relationships.

Herrman and Wallesch (1989) reported from a large study exploring the effects of aphasia on the family context and described substantial changes to the ways in which the aphasic exists within it. In particular, aphasia was found to affect professional, social, psychological and familial issues. Changes were frequently noticed and had an impact on everyday life in relation to acquisition of new tasks for relatives and the fact that relatives had to face new problems. Intermittent changes were reported in several areas, including new tensions and conflicts, aggression towards the patient, parent–child relationships, education and depressive episodes of family members. That is, these changes were sufficiently substantial to affect the daily functioning of the family.

The family of the person with head injury

The predicament of the family where one member suffers a closed head injury is well documented. For the sufferer the problems can range from cognitive, emotional and physical handicaps which may remain with the individual for the rest of his or her life. Given the huge technological development in life-saving techniques, many people with head injury will be saved but bear the burden of a drastically reduced quality of life. This reduction in quality of life has distressing implications for the family members. Social and psychological changes may be forced upon the family at an individual level and at the level of how the family functions as a whole. The interpersonal relationships of the whole family will change initially in response to the immediate impact, and then subsequently as the head-injured person moves towards recovery or some stabilisation period.

The typical profile of the closed head-injured person is commonly under discussion. There is some debate as to whether the condition of the person is attributable to the sequelae of the injury or to the kind of person who became head-injured. Gender is particularly important. For example, males are much more prone to accidents generally in youth and childhood than are females. A substantial number of head injuries come from motor-cycle accidents and the majority of motorcyclists are men. Age is also a factor. People can ride motorcycles at an earlier age than they can drive cars (16 years) and embedded in this is the issue of lack of experience about negotiating roads. There are clear examples of this in insurance cover where far larger sums of money have to be paid out to insure a young rider than a middle-aged rider. Thus, as the profile of the closed head-injured patient can be defined to some extent, so too does the profile of the family become identifiable. The young head-injured patient is likely to still be living with parents and so the issues become related to how the family copes with the return to dependency of a son or daughter who had been expected to emerge as an independent adult within the next few years.

Rollin (1987) discusses the family in terms of a grief response where each member has to move through the transitional stages of grief towards final acceptance of the situation. Various authors refer to the extended denial phase observed in families (Romano 1974) particularly if the head-injured person remains unconscious for some while. The 'sleeping beauty' syndrome is often referred to, where the family's belief focuses on the idea of the unconscious person regaining consciousness and returning to a completely normal pre-morbid existence. Of course, if this does not happen the family may have delayed any realistic emotional response (such as learning to accept the idea of their loved one having special diffi-culties) and find moving towards acceptance even more difficult. However, as Rollin points out, the understanding of this emotional response is complicated. Arguably all families need denial in the early stages in order to keep the family equilibrium on track. What Rollin is concerned about is how long denial can go before it becomes 'abnormal' or 'pathological' and an issue for professional concern. Families may also demonstrate anger towards the medical staff who are trying to help; for example, believing that staff are deliberately withholding information about the patient's recovery is reported. This is related particularly to denial again and to the belief that there is a chance of a perfect recovery – the belief then is that the medical staff are keeping this from the relatives. Romano refers to relatives who take a maladaptive position towards the medical staff demonstrating the following attitude: 'We do not want to talk to you unless you tell us that he will be his old self, just as he was before this accident' (p. 3).

The head injury interrupts the life course and can affect the transitional state of moving from adolescence to adulthood (see Chapter 3). Commonly, the main caretaker of a young head-injured person is the mother or a young spouse or partner. The patient is thrown back on to these people just at the threshold of setting up an independent life, and all parties may experience considerable distress about this. If the head-injured patient already has a relationship with a partner, this needs to be taken into account in considering the recovery profile. As so many are young, there may be associated excess alcohol intake with the accident. The patient may already have established himself as an impulsive person, and thus the pre-morbid personality and relationships may be indicative of responses to rehabilitation. If the head-injured patient has become more moody, possibly aggressive or disinhibited as the result of the injury, then a young partner may suffer greatly in attempting to cope with the loss of 'old' person and learning to cope with the 'new' person.

Rollin discusses several studies which report social isolation, depression and sexual dissatisfaction in wives of brain injured servicemen. Often the head-injured patient becomes emotionally regressed, childlike and overdemanding, and this becomes a drain on the partner's emotional resources. Sexual dysfunction is also reported. This may take the form of lack of sensitivity to the partner's needs, sexual disinterest or sexual preoccupation. In relation to the prospects for the future relationship between the two young people, Rollin defines various critical factors:

>]) the degree of personality and behavioural change in the victim, 2) pre-morbid marital relationship, 3) the spouse's attitude and level of support, 4) level of support for both victim and spouse from members of the extended family, 5) the degree and quality of formal rehabilitation efforts with particular emphasis on family counselling or therapy' (1987, p. 91).

If there are children in the family then their coping abilities may tend to get overlooked. The social isolation that may occur as the result of the changed family status may affect their development. The unaffected partner may use up so much energy on caring for the head-injured person that there is little time left to attend to the needs of the children. The child's personal distress may emerge in the form of behavioural difficulties, truancy, behaviour problems at school and general lack of commitment to the family situation. Older children may leave home earlier than expected in order to avoid the family distress.

Head and neck cancer

There are recognised psychosocial effects of head and neck cancer and the effects of this upon the family. As well as problems with swallowing and chewing there may be significant speech problems which can cause deterioration in communication between family members. The family members may experience great difficulty in communicating and thus become frustrated. Potentially, the family may become socially isolated with a resulting loss of self-esteem and depression.

In an extensive review of the literature on the psychosocial effects, Pruyn et al. (1986) note the family difficulties in people who are laryngectomees. Between 8 and 33 per cent of the laryngectomees reviewed reported that sexual intercourse decreased or was terminated as a consequence of treatment. Darvill (1983) had noted that if a couple's sexual relationship had been satisfactory before then they could be counselled so that it could adjust to the post-operative situation. The most frequent sources of difficulty reported by Darvill are a needless fear of suffocation, egressive air from the stoma and occasional breath odour. Embarrassment about physical appearance is often cited as a reason for cessation of sexual relations, although this could be responsive to counselling.

Darvill notes the importance of a spouse's role in the adjustment of the laryngectomy patient. The spouse may feel the need to be brave in the face of the partner's cancer, but experience great personal fear and threat at the same time. The difficulty about rehabilitation in the laryngectomy situation is that both spouse and patient have to cope with the threat of returning cancer as well as the challenge of rehabilitation. Both need support. There is the potential loss of employment and financial support for both to deal with as well as the difficulties of coping in society where the technicalities of oesophageal speech are not generally understood. Unlike the aphasic speaker, the laryngectomy speaker is very certain about what he or she wishes to say and feels extreme frustration at the difficulties present in doing so.

Female patients who undergo this operation experience particular difficulties about physical appearance and Darvill (1983) confirms the psychological problems associated with this, including difficulties in accepting their own attempts at oesophageal speech.

Issues about communication for families of the elderly person

The normal elderly person (that is, who has no specific communication disorder but has physical and behavioural changes associated with normal ageing) can still find communication problematic. The family constellation can provide essential communicative support for the elderly person socially and for more critical needs. The older generation still, for the most part, think in terms of generations of family members, with traditional spouses, adult children and grandchildren and it is frequently for these people that the elderly person turns for important aspects of communication. The family unit may be critical for the ageing person for a substantial number of elderly people live in the community with either a spouse for support or an adult child – usually a daughter – who provides essential everyday requirements if the elderly person is frail or sick. Given the increasing numbers of elderly people, this generation will need substantial support from health care services, although it is recognised that many families take up the burden of care for their elderly and carry this without any support from the community.

Lubinski and Welland (1997) report the results of research on family members and communicative capacity. The nature and success of communication between elderly spouses has been explored and Sillars and Zietlow (1993) report that from a study of 77 couples (age range 23–83 years) couples were non-committal when discussing conflicts, and expressed interdependence through the use of communal themes and common frames of reference, for example frequently using 'we' pronouns. Shadden (1988) investigated communication between adult children and their elderly parents: the children reported their parents' communicative content as rambling, digressive, repetitive and over-reliant on the past as a topic. Occasional word-finding problems were also reported. Other issues included speech which had become slower, more laboured and affected by hearing loss. The authors state that those children who reported such negative aspects to their parents' speech were also more likely to report poor relationships with their parents, including a difficulty in expression of feeling. This same study examined what adjustments children made towards communicating with their parents; these included speaking louder and simplifying what they said. Studies have also been conducted into how grandchildren and grandparents communicate with each other. Results from a number of studies showed that adult children tended to use a more deferential style towards their grandparents than towards their own parents and also be more congenial. Lubinski and Wellend suggest this is because of the stereotypical view of elderly people and the tendency for over-accommodating speech because of cultural expectations.

The family and the child with a communication impairment

The family has already been shown to be critical in a child's development. However, this becomes more complicated when a child has communication problems. Families are used to dealing with acute short-term problems like colds, or even conditions that require short-term hospitalisation. Minor accidents do happen to children, for example, falling off chairs, tripping over toys. They are part of general expectations about family life. When, however, the child has chronic difficulties such as slow development of communication skill, the family situation is different. Frequently the problems will not be immediately understandable and interactions with the child may begin to be problematic from an early stage. Law and Elias (1996) refer to the differing expectations that families with varying cultural backgrounds may have about developmental aspects in their children. What is assumed to be 'normal' in one family may not be perceived that way in another. Clearly, family communicative behaviour and social environment will have an effect on the child's developing speech and language, which may be to the good of the child or cause problems. There is certainly evidence to indicate that some speech and language problems are familial (for example, stuttering). Law and Elias note that a family history of speech and language problems may be unrecognised until the a child of the youngest generation is referred for help; that may be because the problems were not as severe (but still present) in other generations. Anecdotal report is often referred to in children with Asberger's syndrome where the father may be reported as having some socioprag-matic difficulties which were never previously noticed or diagnosed.

Law and Elias report a survey in which the effects of having a child diagnosed with a speech and language problem varied from parents certain that it had not had adverse effects upon family life to parents who described themselves as devastated at finding that they did not have a 'perfect' child, and who were desperately seeking reasons for why the problem had occurred, including self-blame. Most parents will go through a phase of uncertainty about what sort and extent of a problem their child may have. Although many parents intuitively know that their child has a problem it will take time for professional diagnosis to be complete.

The reactions of siblings to a child with a communication handicap is not well developed in speech and language therapy literature. However, it is clearly a sensitive issue for a family; the risk of excluding the sibling while focusing attention on the child with the handicap is well developed in the general handicap literature, and we need to understand it better in communication handicap. Families need to avoid the secondary problem of the 'silent identified patient' which the sibling(s) may become (Rollin 1987).

Can we say that the effects upon families are similar regardless of the different types of developmental communication impairments which exist? There must surely be some differences between the way a family copes with a child who has a phonological problem and the way we anticipate that a family copes with and reacts to a child with a potential stuttering difficulty. Typically we view the case of a child with a non-fluency problem as being one where the family may influence the outcome of the communication impairment. Hayhow and Levy (1989, p. 51) justify the importance of working with the family of a child with potential stutter by stating that:

- the child's communication skills develop within the context of the family and so the family interaction has a profound effect on how these skills develop

- the major part of the child's communication with adults occurs within the family. Usually talking to adults is more difficult for the child than talking to peers
- the significance that the problem has for the family as a whole and for each member personally can be understood by meeting them all. This should help to identify how the problem with speaking fits into the family's structure and construing
- observation of patterns of interaction and the quality of communication will identify some of the causal and maintaining factors.

The importance of the family in this context is further confirmed by the therapeutic guidelines reported by Hayhow and Levy which focus specifically on family relationships and take the attention on the problem away from the speech of the child. Although not all approaches to therapy for children with non-fluency follow this approach exactly, the basic philosophy for non-fluency in children is to incorporate the family relationship into management and treatment. In their work on how to help the child and family with potential stuttering, Hayhow and Levy provide a firm set of guidelines based upon the view that working with the family is critical to outcome. These guidelines include evaluation of the family with a recommendation that two therapists are involved, helping the family to construct a family tree including three generations as a way of helping the family to focus their attention on their own history, and exploring the family construct system.

Rustin (1991) investigated the influence of the family context upon the development of stuttering in childhood. In an extensive survey of 209 completed case histories, the overall conclusion demonstrated that the dysfluent children in the study had much higher problem rates individually and within their family than would be expected for children of similar age and background.

Rollin (1987) discusses the role of the family in relation to the child with emerging language disorder. If language develops in the context of interaction with family members, then clearly there must be implications for that emergence of language if there is dysfunction within the family and poor communication. There is very little information on this subject, but there are certainly many questions to explore. Although professionals recognise the importance of a good communicative environment for developing language in young children, we do not have detailed understanding of what relationship this environment has with language. It is not straightforward. If family dysfunction and poor interaction between members was a true causative factor, then all children born into dysfunctional families would have language problems. This is clearly not the case. The relationship is not that simple.

Is there any way in which we can identify what specific effects a language impairment may have on family relationships? Rollin draws attention to what can happen if the parent has difficulty in interpreting the child's immature language use. If the parent shows non-comprehension, then the child may feel rejected and be more reluctant to communicate. In time this has repercussions all family members and the psychological ease within the family may get increasingly disturbed.

The research on maternal communication with the infant is well researched, but takes a different position. It looks at the two-way communicative relationship and thus takes out the whole family system. It may be possible for example for the mother–child communicative process to be strong and positive enough to facilitate good practice of communication, but still exist within a family unit which functions poorly. As Duck (1986) comments, so much of the research into families is not specifically about family systems, but more about focus on parts of families, such as mother–child interaction. Conti-Ramsden and Dykins (1991) were able to show that parental styles, in particular maternal styles of interaction, are consistent within a family. Factors such as number of turns in the interaction were consistent characteristics between mother and their children of the same language stage, regardless of whether there was language delay. Although this form of research into communicative styles varies from investigations into psychological interaction, what could be explored further is the importance of turn taking forming an emotional and relationship standpoint. That is, is consistent turn taking any sort of marker for good relationships?

Finally in this section we need to examine the ways in which a phonological or speech impairment can affect the family. We have little evidence here, but clinically it is well recognised that parents and other family members have difficulties in coping with a child who may be unintelligible for a variety of reasons. If the family are embarrassed by the child's speech or anxious about the future, this will affect the child's interpretation of being in a family and of what having close relationships means. We do not have much information on the long-term effects of speech impairment, but an example can be located in work by Syder (1998) who discusses James, a young man who attended electropalatography therapy for help with intransigent lateralisation of sibilant fricatives and affricates. During this experience James was identified as needing help with relationships and he was able to gain the services of a speech and language therapist who was also a counsellor. During the course of the counselling it emerged that no family discussion had ever taken place about James's speech difficulties, that James recalled being teased at school and having a mother who was overcritical and denigratory. His father, to whom he was close, had died when James was in his teens. As an adult this young man reported shyness, loneliness, a failure to make relationships with women even though he wanted to, and overall low self-esteem. Although it would be unrealistic to attribute all of these problems to his speech, there is certainly an issue to do with the family function and the way in which James's speech problems were handled.

The family and the deaf child

Following on from an initial large-scale study into the impact of deafness on young children, Gregory, Bishop and Sheldon (1995) were able to contact 91 of the original 122 families eighteen years later to investigate what had happened to them in the intervening years. In this huge survey – which looked at family life, education, being deaf in a hearing world and relationships – what was very clear was the effect that difficulty with communication had on the lives of all the family members. In the original report 76 per cent of the parents had described their main problem with their child to be communication. Eighteen years later over half of the parents still claimed to be critically concerned with their child's communication skills. At this later stage the parents had reflected on the importance of communication and had learnt it as a conscious skill to be attained rather than the unconscious spontaneous development which exists in most hearing families. Many of the parents claimed that they made deliberate attempts to include their children in family conversations, but that they had to use strategies to do this, such as frequently turning to check if their child had understood. In many families where the deaf child had severe difficulties, the person who was most successful at communicating with the child was the mother. In other families communication was described as being better with one family member, and this too was frequently the mother. Many of the parents stated that they felt the communicative difficulties hampered not only the everyday dialogue between family members but also influenced self-esteem and the development of confidence and identity. If the deaf child or young person could not hear all details of family events and associated problems it meant that he or she did not feel a complete member of the family unit. This had deleterious effects. In this particular sample not all families had been given the opportunity for learning sign language, as their children had grown up in a time when oral language was seen as a crucial skill to learn. Consequently many had failed but had not learnt the alternative skill of signing as compensation.

The effect on the child who is severely deprived

The importance of the environment for the development of communication is well documented and uncontroversial nowadays (Locke 1993). But we have evidence from other sources which gives us a perspective on what happens if a child is reared or exists in a completely deprived environment. Because of the recent attention upon Romanian orphanages and the plight of those children, researchers have been able to revisit what is known about deprivation and examine the implications of this again. There are some extreme conditions reported. The reports from the orphanages when they were made public showed children surviving in severe deprivation. McMullan and Fisher (1992) described approximately

30 children in a room where there was complete silence, the children spending 20 out of 24 hours in their cribs, often rocking back and forth on their hands and knees or shifting from foot to foot while standing up in them. The caretaker to child ratio for infants and toddlers ranged from 1:10 to 1:20 and little interaction took place between the child and the caretaker. As well as impoverished social interaction, the children were not encouraged to develop eating skills. Children up to two-and-a-half years of age were described as taking food only from a bottle. This feature is reported in other work which has demonstrated the effects of poor eating. Groze and Ileana (1996) who followed up children adopted in North America from Romanian orphanages found the children had been undernourished and when placed in a family environment had begun to overeat, as if they had never learnt to recognise the feeling of being full. Groze and Ileana (1996) demonstrate that the length of time in institution-alised care was significantly related to the adoptive parents' reports of pounds below weight at placement, inches below normal height, delay in fine and gross motor skills and delay in the development of language skills. The authors point out, however, that this does not necessarily imply that the delays were only due to institutionalisation; these children might have already been delayed when placed in the institutions.

In Romania, the orphanages were supposed to represent state-organised care, but in some societies there is no such care and children may be left to develop without any support at all. Some of the cases are deeply shocking. Bartlett and Limsila (1992) report the case of Mai, a 3-and-a-half-year-old girl incarcerated in a bamboo cage in a village in Thailand, after it was feared that she had contracted rabies. Six years later, when she was released, she had lost almost all motor control, was incontinent, had grand mal epilepsy and was without speech (in spite of normal speech development being reported by the her parents at the time of her incarceration).

Findings also suggest that psychosocial deprivation has a more profound effect upon verbal rather than visuospatial skills. McNeil, Polloway and Smith (1984) reviewed the cases of 56 children who had been reported as severely deprived and of whom 36 had either no speech or no intelligible speech when found. What the authors state is that the real reasons for their lack of speech were never extrapolated because society did not have the diagnostic tools. As the authors comment, severe environmental deprivation may have been the cause, but importantly it had occurred at the critical period for language learning; or that the children who were deprived were learning disabled or autistic and this condition had gone unrecognised. Certainly some evidence shows that children who are taken out of the impoverished environment and given a stable home often improve extremely quickly – an often-quoted example of this is the twins described by Koluchova (1972) who were eventually removed from extreme cruelty and neglect at the age of 7 and who caught up with normal development rapidly, thus reversing the effects of the deprivation.

As research in this area continues, the international expertise on adoption and institutional effects will be become more and more sophisticated. Also, as Skuse (1984) suggests, analysis of effects of severe deprivation is providing an experimental paradigm from which we can understand more about developmental problems in children who have normal environments but still show delays or abnormalities. Are there critical periods in development where deprivation makes a permanent difference, and are there periods where minimal stimulation has no permanent effect?

What help is there?

We have seen many aspects of family life by looking at all the different factors included in this chapter. Families are at best nurturing, loving units where a child can thrive and an adult can be supported in a time of crisis, or at worst a unit in which a child fails and an adult cannot cope. One of the ways in which families can be helped is by means of therapy, and this is an approach which has become more widely accepted during the last decade in Great Britain.

Family therapy

This approach aims to produce change in the family system as a way of helping the family cope more productively with problems. In essence, the family needs to be able to develop new ways of understanding and dealing with situations in order to permit the development of new and more useful behaviours. Winter (1992) discusses the personal construct theory approach to family therapy where the therapist needs to elicit the systematic understanding of individual and whole family construct systems. That is, as the individual has a construct system, so too have family members as a group, demonstrating that they have what Epting (1984) terms a 'shared meaning' which constitutes a family construct system. This family construct system governs how the family operates so that the family interaction is structured around the way the family sees its reality represented by a construct system. If, for example, that system is very hierarchical and rigid, then coping with change may be difficult because the family cannot deal with any thing which poses a threat to the construct system. As a way of eliciting change one approach is for family members to watch each other being interviewed on video tape. Shared constructs are then identified from the tapes and brought up for discussion, first as a way of defining the family and then for elaborating the construing and developing an understanding of the alternative.

Mancuso and Handin (1980) developed an approach to family therapy working on parenting skills. Parents are asked to consider their own constructs relating to parenting and the constructions of their children, and if necessary reconstruct their parenting roles. The aim is to enable the parent to acknowledge and understand that there may be differences in the way they and their children construe events and reflect this under-standing in the way they behave towards their children in the future. Hayhow and Levy (1989) report the use of personal construct family therapy in relation to the family of a child with emerging stuttering. For example, an exploration of whether either of the parents construes dysfluent speech negatively is important for the therapist to know. Also, the family view of the problem is of value. How does the family construe the stuttering? Is it viewed as something that is a health issue, or an individual negative attribute which needs to be got rid of? Frequently families perceive stuttering as a form of laziness about speaking. Any of these constructions can have problematic effects upon the child and it is therefore critical for the therapist to gain this understanding by exploring the construct systems of family members and the whole group. Hayhow and Levy describe the potential problems if the stuttering child is viewed negatively compared with other children in the family. Their evidence suggests that this is most critical when there is a stuttering brother and a 'good' fluent sister. The fluent sister may be seen as better behaved and altogether more reasonable than the brother and the polarisation of the two may increase in extremity as time goes on, unless the therapist draws attention to it. Hayhow and Levy also indicate that other family members, or those close to it, may contribute to the positioning of the stuttering child, such as grandparents or even teachers.

Family therapy for families affected by illness or disability has to include time spent on defining the illness and what it means to each individual, and a consideration of other factors influencing the family at present (for example, the family may be coping with a child who has suffered a head injury but also be travelling to visit a sick parent in another town every week). Family therapists also need to ensure that the family take responsi-bility for the situation rather than allowing it to become a professional problem. Altschuler (1997) discusses the ideas around 'normalising' an illness; that is helping the family see that the illness or handicap is a part of their family functioning but not all of it, and that neglecting the needs of other members may lead to future problems. It may also be necessary for the family to acknowledge the needs of the sick person and the therapist needs to bring this out during the therapeutic process.

Wahrborg (1991, p. 81) reviewed family therapy with aphasic speakers and described the following aims for therapy.

1 To explore cognitive and emotional patterns of the family before, during and after onset of aphasia in a family member.
2 To teach the family about the handicap and common reactions associ-ated with it.

3 To encourage and reinforce emotional sharing in the family and guide its members in the process of acting out grief, anger, frustration, etc.

4 To bring up common issues faced in these families and introduce open and direct communication on delicate topics such as sexuality, bodily changes, etc.

5 To encourage the aphasic family to explain what kind of help he or she wants from the other members of the family, such as if and when they want help with verbal cueing.

6 To teach the family how to time their interactions differently.

7 To teach family members to notice non-verbal communication behaviour, especially emotional qualities, and to check and clarify their interpretations.

8 To teach special feedback techniques if the aphasic family member suffers from apraxia, impaired control of affect or impaired motivation.

9 To recommend to the family to refrain from formal linguistic training of the aphasic speaker unless they have been specifically asked to by the speech pathologist.

Wahrborg argues that the special needs of the aphasic speaker make the running of a family therapy group much more bound to rules and structure. That is, reliance on general approaches to therapy may have to be modified because of the communication aspects which may attention to as well. Wahrborg also describes the different phases of therapy, the social phase involving getting to know the family; the explorative phase, exploring communication potential and possibilities within the family; the problem orienting phase, where individual members are interviewed and issues identified. After this, the therapist can reach the diagnostic phase and the procedure is completed by the therapeutic phase where one problem is highlighted and worked through in therapy.

Nicholls, Varchevker and Pring (1996) explored the use of family therapy with aphasic speakers when the therapy is conducted jointly by a family therapist and a speech and language therapist. The personal questionnaire rapid scaling technique (PQRST, Mulhall 1978) was used as a means of identifying change. Two families were used in this project and positive changes were found for both, although the changes were stronger with the aphasic speaker than for the other family members. Also, changes were more marked in the time following therapy rather than during the period of therapy. There is the possibility that any sort of psychological change takes time to be evident and this is why the changes were more obvious later on.

Conclusion

Communication impairments affect family functioning and families affect the person with the communication impairment. Often we underestimate the impact this has on improvement and recovery rates. All that we know about attitudes and self-knowledge forms part of the interplay of families, whatever their structure. Professionals have to be able recognise the multi-faceted aspect of the individual with a communication handicap and its position with the family context and background in order to deal most appropriately with any remedial problem.

The question also arises about the role of the speech and language therapist in relation to work with families. Is it sufficient only to know about these matters, or do direct skills in family work need to be acquired? This may be worked out more formally in the next decade of speech and language therapy practice, but for the present, those who work with families develop those skills with experience. What we need to do now is develop a clearer literature upon what effects communication impairment has directly upon the family, what role the family has upon the develop-ment and maintenance of an impairment, and what more we can add to intervention to enhance the outcome of therapy using the family as a route for change.

Exercises

What are families for?

The following is the response of an 11-year-old girl to the question, 'What are families for?'

> Mummies and daddies are meant for looking after you. Buying you presents at Christmas. If you take chores in turn there are more of you to do it if you are in a family. To care for each other. Adults have an excuse to watch children's television programmes. Adults buy you clothes and boss you about. Families are for explaining things to children. If you have parents they tell you extra stuff if you are in a family.

What purpose did your family serve for you when you were a child? Can you recall any specific examples of being aware that you were a part of a family?

What is good and bad about being a child?

The following are the statements of a 9-year-old girl in response to the question, 'What is good and bad about being a child?'

> *Bad about being a child*
>   You get bossed around a lot.
>   You have to go to school.
>   You can't have things other people don't like.
> *Good about being a child*
>   You go to birthday parties.

You go on holiday.
If something goes wrong you always have somebody to tell.
You get bought lots of clothes.

Do children generally reflect on what it means to be a child? Would you expect a complicated answer? If you have children in your acquaintance, find out their response to the same question.

Recommended reading

Altschuler J (1997) Working with Chronic Illness. London: Macmillan.

Hoen B, Thelander M, Worsley J (1997) Improvement in psychological well-being of people with aphasia and their families: evaluation of a community-based programme. Aphasiology 11(7): 681–91.

Chapter 5
Psychology in the Health Care Setting

Overview

This chapter will enable you to:

- understand the psychological meaning of health and illness
- gain an understanding of models of health and the ways in which people respond to health care
- look at specific examples of health care as they relate to the situation of speech and language handicapped people.

Introduction

- Your uncle has had a mild heart attack at the age of 54. His doctor has told him that he must eat a more healthy diet. Because he works occasional night shifts in a busy factory his eating patterns vary from day to day. Sometimes he is very busy and can only rush into the canteen and eat a greasy meal of chips with something. He smokes too, and has found it impossible to give up.

  The doctor has given him some advice, which, with medication, may contribute to a much healthier and more positive future. The solution is given to your uncle.

  Five months later your uncle has been unable to alter his diet or give up smoking. Can you think of an explanation for this?

- You are 20 years old and female. Since going to university you have enjoyed a good social life but you have always been slightly overweight and now want to try to lose some pounds. Today you wake up and hate the way you look. If you were thinner you would be able to wear the clothes you really liked. You decide that you will start to diet immediately.

  At eight o'clock that evening you find yourself in the kitchen eating choco-late biscuits. Can you think of an explanation for this?

As can be seen from the two examples above, there may be medical or cultural reasons why health behaviour must be changed, but the success of these attempts may vary from individual to individual and may be due, not to physical or medical reasons – but to psychological causes.

The interface between health and psychological reactions has been demonstrated to be critical. This chapter will look at the psychological aspects of health; how the individual's psychological understanding may affect responses to treatment, and what factors are involved in good or bad health behaviour.

But before these can be further discussed, we need to be clear about what we mean by 'health'. What is it? Are you healthy if you are not dying of a progressive disease? Are you healthy only if you keep fit by running regularly and eating a restricted diet? Are all non-smokers healthy people? The ways in which health is defined and understood can critically influence not only health care on an individual basis but also government planning policies.

The World Health Organisation (1948) defined health as being 'a complete state of physical, mental and social well-being and not merely the absence of disease or infirmity'. In 1984, a further definition was provided:

> Health is the extent to which an individual or group is able, on the one hand, to realise aspirations and satisfy needs; and on the other hand, to change or cope with the environment. Health is, therefore, seen as a resource for everyday life, not the object of living; it is a positive concept emphasising social and personal resources, as well as physical capacities.

This is an ambitious view of health. We are lucky people if we can maintain physical, mental and social wellbeing throughout our lives.

Most of us have excursions into ill health in some form or other. If we are lucky, we recover, but, of course, some people do not. Why people vary in their vulnerability to illness is a multifaceted issue and has been substantially researched. It is has been established, for example, that health status varies across social groups. Although the reasons why this occurs are complex (see Alder 1995), there is a definite trend for the most unhealthy people to be at the lower end of the social scale. Whether there is a direct relationship between income and health status however is not clear cut because genetic factors also affect this, as do cultural traditions – health-related behaviours differ between cultural groups. Life events too, may affect health status. They can precede physical or psychological health problems and can trigger or exacerbate psychological disorders. Many patients can explain the onset of their stroke in relation to a major life stress preceding the stroke. Similarly, environmental conditions can affect health. The development of better housing (for most people) during this century and the improvement of hygiene and immunisation programmes have resulted in a more healthy society in Britain; however, unemployment is associated with poor health. Unfortunately, the association works in both directions. Being unemployed can be shown to have an adverse effect on health status, while the person in poor health will have less chance of gaining employment.

Thus we can have an understanding of factors which affect health status. However, health is also affected by the individual's behaviour – it is not only external factors which influence it. Frequently the behaviour of the individual causes more or less likelihood of illness and this has to be taken into account in the equation.

Kasl and Cobb (1966), in a frequently quoted article, refer to health behaviour as 'any activity undertaken by a person believing himself to be healthy for the purpose of preventing disease or detecting it at an asymptomatic stage' (p. 118). An example of this would be taking up a regular exercise programme. In the field of communication impairment an example would be the public speaker who developed and maintained good vocal habits in order to avoid dysphonia.

As a contrast, illness behaviour can be defined as 'any activity undertaken by a person who feels ill, to define the state of his health and discover a suitable remedy' (p. 118). Here the illness behaviour would be seeking out help from the GP or purchasing medication from the chemist for relief of symptoms, or the public speaker who was required to seek out GP advice because of loss of voice.

Sick role behaviour is defined as an activity carried out specifically for the purpose of getting well and would include attending for voice therapy if dysphonia had resulted from excessive vocal abuse.

Many of the health problems of modern societies relate to chronic illness associated with cancer, heart disease and cerebrovascular disease, and much of the medical care in these illnesses is concerned with long-term care as opposed to short-term acute care. Coping with disability is an issue for the individual as well as for those who make economic and social policies about the community. In addition it has been recognised that modifications to behaviour can affect the amount of medical care required. For example, in our first example at the beginning of the chapter, the man may avoid any more heart disease if he radically alters his lifestyle. The success of altering his lifestyle will depend on psychological factors as much as anything else.

Psychological effects play a different role in the range of conditions which may occur (Banyard 1996):

- there may be an interaction between the symptom(s) and the individual's psychology (e.g. pain, menstrual problems)
- there may be conditions which occur because of a faulty psychological approach to situations (e.g. smoking or drinking to relieve anxiety)
- a medical condition may cause psychological distress (e.g. an acute illnesses or an accident resulting in head injury).

All of these aspects can affect our clients directly or indirectly.

Health belief model

This model has been used in a large number of studies of health protective behaviour and was originally developed by Rosenstock (1966). According to the model an individual's readiness to take health action is determined by four main factors:

- the perceived susceptibility to the disease
- the perceived severity or seriousness of the disease
- the perceived benefits of the health action
- the perceived barriers to performing the action.

This therefore describes the influence of individual belief on health behaviour. This looks at the reasons why an individual decides to carry out health behaviour and is related to the concept of susceptibility. For example, a woman with close relatives who have died of cancer may make an informed decision not to smoke because of perceived susceptibility to the disease. Similarly, a public speaker may avoid shouting, drinking spirits and talking with a laryngeal infection because of perceived susceptibility to loss of voice, whereas a person without a public speaking role may not see these factors as contributing to the health status of the voice.

Also, health behaviour is affected by the individual's perception of the severity of the condition. One individual may agree to eat a low-fat diet because of the severe perceived risk of heart disease, whereas another may not keep to such a diet to avoid weight gain because weight gain alone is not viewed as a severe risk.

Another view might be that keeping to a low-fat diet is worthwhile because being slim is a benefit in everyday life. But a perceived barrier to this behaviour could be the prohibitive cost of buying low-fat healthy foods. The health belief model has been applied in many health care contexts, such as cancer studies in women. Ronis and Harel (1989) investigated breast self-examination (BSE) and its relationship to health beliefs. They found that an increase in the perceived benefit of BSE and the perceived susceptibility to breast cancer significantly increased the likelihood of BSE, whereas an increase in the perceived cost (barriers) of BSE significantly reduced the likelihood of practice.

Locus of control

Rotter (1966b) postulated that consistent differences exist with respect to a person's belief in the way his or her behaviour will affect the control of life events. These beliefs are called 'locus of control' and derive from work on social learning theory. A distinction is made between the individual who is 'internal' and the person who is 'external'. The internal person expects reinforcements to follow in direct consequence of a piece of behaviour, thus believing his or her actions to be responsible for outcome. The external person perceives behaviour to be directed by external factors such as chance, fate, society's influence and so on. Of course the terms 'internal' and 'external' are not meant to imply that a person is entirely one way or the other. As Lefcourt (1976) suggests, the perception of control is a process where the individual becomes engaged in the process developing an expectancy regarding causation. The terms reflect the individual's most common tendency, therefore, to expect events to be contingent or not upon actions.

The theory of locus of control has been extensively explored and has applications in many branches of health psychology. For example, it may affect a client's expectations about therapy and also the client's potential success in therapy. Foon (1987) reviews the literature on the use of locus of control as a variable in explaining outcome following psychotherapy. The conclusions state the importance of determining locus of control in clients before deciding upon a particular therapeutic model, and that therapists should be aware of their own control orientations as this may affect therapeutic success.

Partridge and Johnston (1989) developed a recovery locus of control (RLOC) scale to explore the beliefs of people suffering stroke and wrist fracture. In both groups using the RLOC pre- and post-rehabilitation, greater internality was associated with faster recovery. The implications from this study are again that health care approaches will be more successful if tailored to the beliefs of the individual patient.

Because of the importance of recognising feelings and reactions to being aphasic and the limited exploration of these so far in the literature, it was decided to investigate these in a small group intervention study and this is described below. So far very little work has been done on the way in which the individual's belief system could affect the rehabilitation of the aphasic speaker. Brumfitt and Sheeran (1997) evaluated a group therapy intervention conducted with six aphasic speakers. Measures included the use of an application of the locus of improvement scale (Partridge and Johnston 1996). Evidence was found to show that stronger beliefs about the role of personal effort in improving speech were predictive of improvements in communication attitudes. The recovery locus of control scale (RLOC) is a nine-item scale which measures two factors: beliefs about the role of self in the process of recovery (internal beliefs) and beliefs about the role of external factors in recovery (external beliefs). The scale has satisfactory reliability and has been shown to be predictive of behavioural outcomes in health settings. Five items are used to measure internal beliefs (e.g. 'Improving my speech is a matter of my own determination rather than anything else') and four items are used to measure external beliefs (e.g. 'My own contribution to my improvement in my speech doesn't amount to much'). Four of the items on the scale were altered slightly: the term 'recovery' was changed to 'improvement in my speech' in order to make the scale relevant to this client group. An example of the scale is presented in Figure 5.1.

Internal Items

How I manage in the future depends on me not on what other people can do for me.
   Strongly agree   Agree   In between   Disagree   Strongly disagree

It's what I do to help myself that's really going to make all the difference.
   Strongly agree   Agree   In between   Disagree   Strongly disagree

It's up to me to make sure I make the best recovery possible under the circumstances.
   Strongly agree   Agree   In between   Disagree   Strongly disagree

Getting better now is a matter of my own determination rather than anything else.
   Strongly agree   Agree   In between   Disagree   Strongly disagree

It doesn't matter how much help you get – in the end it's your own efforts that count.
   Strongly agree   Agree   In between   Disagree   Strongly disagree

External Items

It's often best just to wait and see what happens.
   Strongly agree   Agree   In between   Disagree   Strongly disagree

My own efforts are not very important, my recovery really depends on others.
   Strongly agree   Agree   In between   Disagree   Strongly disagree

My own contribution to my recovery doesn't amount to much.
   Strongly agree   Agree   In between   Disagree   Strongly disagree

I have little or no control over my progress from now on.
   Strongly agree   Agree   In between   Disagree   Strongly disagree

Figure 5.1. Recovery locus of control
Source: Partridge and Johnston 1989.

This is an interesting use of the locus of control concept. It is, of course, dependent on the respondent having sufficient understanding of written language to make use of the scale. The aphasic speakers in Brumfitt and Sheeran's group coped well with the answers but it must be acknowledged that this scale would need modification if applied to people with severe aphasia or other client groups such as those with learning disabilities.

Other work relating to communication disorder has been carried out using the recovery locus of control scale. Interestingly, the relationship between locus of control and stuttering behaviour was explored well before this phenomena was looked at in aphasiology. DeNil and Kroll (1995) explored the relationship between locus of control and long-term stuttering treatment outcome in adult stutterers. Here the study investigated the extent to which adult stutterers' scores on the locus of control behaviour scale were predictive of their ability to maintain speech fluency immediately following intensive treatment and approximately two years on. While most subjects showed a significant long-term improvement in fluency, no predictive relationship was found between scores on the LCB scale and level of fluency. LCB scores were found to be predictive of the subject's fluency self-evaluation measured post-treatment and at follow up. What is important is not necessarily the results. The critical point lies in the fact that it was considered worth looking at and that it demonstrated that self-evaluation and health beliefs have the potential to be entangled with the communication problem itself.

Quality of life

It is well recognised that many medical treatments may save the life of an individual, but have devastating effects upon the quality of that individual's everyday experience. Head-injured people, for example, may be saved from death following a road accident by sophisticated technology, but may live a damaged personal life following this. This raises questions about the purpose of health care. Baum, Gatchel and Kranz (1997) define health care in terms of providing the opportunity to allow people to live for a long time, and also to improve the quality of their lives before death. Of course, quality of life has many definitions but it generally refers to an acceptable level of social and psychological wellbeing. Kaplan and Bush (1982) include a range of dimensions in their description of quality of life:

*   physical symptoms experienced by the patient
*   functional status – their ability to take care of themselves and to conduct activities of daily life
*   role activities – the ability to work at one's job and at home
*   social functioning – including personal interactions and intimacy
*   emotional status – anxiety, stress and depression
*   cognitive level and vitality
*   perceptions of one's own health – the sense of positive wellbeing
*   general satisfaction with life.

From the perspective of delivering health care services, the measurement of quality of life has become an important dimension. Outcome from a specific treatment policy can be measured in terms of the effects upon quality of life. Some debate has taken place regarding the dimensions which should be evaluated in a quality of life evaluation for people suffering stroke. The *Health of the Nation Key Area Handbook* (Department of Health 1993) suggested action to streamline the assessment of people with strokes. These were the development of 'common assessment procedures throughout the rehabilitation process' and a 'standard assessment procedure which could act as the basis of outcome measures, against which performance could be monitored'. Ebrahim, Baer and Nouri (1987) reviewed outcome measures in stroke rehabilitation research and criticised the use of broader measures. There was a recognition that assessing physical recovery and self-care was too limiting and a strong recommendation was made that subjective measures of health status and quality of life should be included in future research. Sarno (1997) refers to the challenges posed in constructing measures of quality of life. These challenges arise because of the difficulty in extrapolating exactly what the construct of quality of life is, and also in applying appropriate methodology to measure it. Sarno refers to self-report measures as being the most commonly used method, with observer ratings also used. However, there is some debate about the differences between the two and whether the subjective self-view extracts the key information or not. Some authors have shown that relatives and health care providers, as judges of the client's quality of life status, have tended to under-rate it.

There is no doubt that quality of life issues in stroke survivors is extremely important because of the devastating effects of stroke upon the individual. Niemi et al. (1988) showed deterioration among several domains of life in 46 stroke survivors under the age of 65 years four years after a stroke. Hemispheric localisation of the lesion, paresis, coordination disturbances and especially tendency to depression were correlated with a deterioration in the quality of life. Sarno (1997) notes that the relationship between quality of life and actual status after stroke is not clear. For example, in one study stroke patients with little or no physical dysfunction reported poor quality of life. In another study patients whose activities of daily living skills were enhanced over a two-year period did not report associated quality of life changes.

Sarno (1997) reported a study of quality of life in 59 consecutively admitted post-stroke aphasic patients who were treated in rehabilitation and followed from three months to twelve months post onset. Results showed that improved quality of life in the first post-stroke year was related to intensity and duration of aphasia rehabilitation services that addressed language, communication strategies, copying skills and psychosocial issues. As Sarno states, the success of rehabilitation must be considered in terms of its impact on the quality of life of the individual. Finding appropriate approaches to aphasic speakers to enhance quality of life has to be done in a health care context that has finite resources.

Compliance: its relationship to health behaviour

This is sometimes called therapeutic cooperation and refers to the behaviour carried out by a patient or client following a consultation with a health professional. If patients are given instructions, they may or may not carry those instructions out. This is commonly recognised in medical consultations when giving instructions for taking prescriptions. Some patients will follow the instructions perfectly while others may not do so at all. Similarly, in speech and language therapy contexts, clients may be given work to do during the week. Parents of children with language disorders may fail to keep up with the practice and so be unhelpful in the child's development.

The type of compliance required may vary according to the behaviour that the person is being asked to do. Banyard (1996) talks about four different types: first, that which asks the patient to take short-term medication; second, that which asks for positive changes to the individual's lifestyle, such as 'take more exercise'; third, that which asks a person to stop a behaviour, such as smoking or eating so much fatty food; and finally that which requires individuals in certain contexts to respond to a long-term treatment regime, such as in the case of diabetes where a specific diet is necessary. Clearly the amount of compliance varies according to the type required, and the long-term commitment of a diabetic diet may be more of a difficult task than short-term medication for flu. However, the issue appears to be more complicated than length of commitment.

Ley (1988), who has written extensively on patient behaviour in relation to health advice, summarised the reasons for non-compliance with drug therapy:

- not taking medicine
- taking too much
- incorrect intervals between doses
- incorrect duration
- taking other medicines in addition
- taking medicines with alcohol

Thus the patient's taking of medication may easily go wrong. Baum et al. (1997) report work which demonstrates that patients' errors in administering medication could account for up to 15 per cent of hospitalisations among the elderly. Errors with medication are also one of the primary reasons for hospitalisations among diabetic children. Similarly the speech and language therapy client may fail to carry out the instructions correctly so that there will be either no effect from the remediation or an identifiable detrimental effect.

If so many people fail to carry out instructions, how might this situation be improved? Is it really possible to determine exactly why an individual is non-compliant and also to develop predictors about this? How can we know who has been non-compliant and who has not? Can we find out just by asking the individual patients? These are all difficult questions in which to find precise answers. Kaplan, Sallis and Patterson (1993) discuss issues about self-reporting of compliance. Patients typically over-report compliance to doctors and this has been shown in conditions where a pill count has also been taken for objective evidence. Studies have also shown that doctors' estimates of compliance tend to be artificially high. However, other studies have shown a reverse situation where patients were accurate in self-reporting – this was shown to be due to situations where the patient clearly understood the condition and instructions.

Reported studies have indicated that aspects of the actual prescription regimen may affect the compliance with the task. Thus if there are unpleasant side effects, or the regimen is too complex or disrupts everyday routine too much, there is a greater chance of non-compliance. Also, personality differences affect compliance. Some people accept advice more readily than others. Social support and family guidance may also affect the compliance, as does educational background. The well-educated, for example, will be more likely to comply because of under-standing the importance of taking medication or following health advice.

Other work has looked at cognitive factors and the way information is presented to people. It has been postulated that people may fail to follow doctors' orders owing to genuine misunderstanding of what they are told. Partly this is affected by the overuse of technical terms, plus the patient's perception of the illness or expectations about it which can affect the individual's interpretation of the information (Korsch, Gozzi and Francis 1968; Roth et al. 1962). Some studies have shown that patients forget the information given to them if it is presented verbally only. Also there is a demonstrated reluctance for patients to ask questions in order to increase their understanding of instructions. Ley (1988) summarised the literature on the individual's memory for medical information. The findings showed that patients generally tend to forget what the doctor tells them and that specific instructions and advice are more likely to be forgotten than other information. The more information a patient is given the more likely he or she will be to forget. Ley reported that patients will remember best what they are told first and what they as individuals consider to be the most important part of the message. Intelligent patients do not appear to remember more than less intelligent ones, neither is there a difference between older and younger patients. Anxiety has been shown to play part in the success in receiving the message, and moderately anxious patients appear to remember information better than those who are highly anxious and those who are not anxious at all.

As a result there have been studies that have looked at the means of enhancing the patient's ability to understand and retain information. Ley, in reviewing these, showed that improved communication and specific information giving could aid recovery and decrease patients' anxiety. Giving the most important information first is advised, as is the style in which the information is presented. Patients must be given information so that the most important instructions are highlighted by the verbal style of the speaker.

An alternative to verbal information is written information. This can be reread at a later date, therefore enhancing memory, and it can be designed so that specific important points can be brought out. Morris and Groft (1982) reviewed a number of studies on this topic and found that the median percentage of patients requesting written information about their medication was 77 per cent. Thus there is evidence that patients are favourably disposed to this. One study looking at women undergoing hysterectomy operations (Young and Humphrey 1985) found that those who received a booklet about how to manage in hospital and cope with anxiety showed less post-operative pain and distress and were discharged from hospital more quickly than controls who did not receive the booklet. Ellis et al. (1979) compared the use of written and oral information on patients who were discharged from a medical and respiratory unit. One group received oral information alone on aspects of their treatment and expectations for prognosis, and the second group received both oral and written information. At a follow-up appointment the group that had received both forms of information demonstrated much better under-standing of their illness than the others.

However, even the application of written information as an aid to under-standing has its difficulties. These relate to the complexity of language, whether the patient is likely to keep the written material for future refer-ence or dispose of it quickly, or store it away and forget about it.

The extent to which written information is understandable has been investigated; the way in which this is usually evaluated is in terms of a readability score which can be applied to how fast a passage can be read, how difficult it is, the probability it will be read and the knowledge of the content following the reading. The SMOG (simple measure of gobblede-gook readability formula, McLaughlin 1969) has been applied in many medical contexts including that of speech and language therapy. It involves calculating the number of words containing three or more sylla-bles in three groups of ten consecutive sentences. A further calculation is obtained taking the square root of this value and adding it to 3, as below.

SMOG rating = 3 + the square root of the polysyllabic count

Other readability formulae are also available, such as Flesch (1948). Ley (1988) reports that these correlate well with each other. The SMOG rating was used to assess the level of the material presented in several published booklets available for aphasic speakers and their partners. As an example, *The Psychological Effects of Stroke – a Guide to the Carer*, published by the Stroke Association, was scored with a readability score of 11, indicating that it is accessible to most of the population. The College of Speech and Language Therapists' booklet, *Aphasia-communication Disorder Following Brain Damage*, had a score of 13, indicating that that the reader would have to have attained 'A' level standard at least to under-stand the material.

Brumfitt, Atkinson and Greated (1994) explored the responses of carers of aphasic speakers to a written information booklet, which had been given a SMOG rating of 9. Fourteen carers of aphasic speakers agreed to receive the booklet and keep it for three months. Each carer was given this at the point of discharge from inpatient acute hospital care. The carers were then followed up and interviewed and completed a questionnaire, which explored the carer's view on the quality of information supplied about stroke and about speech symptoms. It also explored the carer's subjective feelings about the booklet. The qualitative results indicated that although the carers were appreciative of the booklet, 42 per cent reported that it had not provided new information. Of interest, 77 per cent went back to read the booklet again, a small number read it once and the same 77 per cent reported that they kept returning to it for reference. There was no clear agreement about the method of information. Approximately one-third of the carers agreed it was better to have written information, one-third preferred the oral route and one-third reported a preference for both presentations. Clearly further work needs to be done in this area.

Social factors in health care for the chronically ill or disabled

Consequences of disease have been conceptualised by the International classification of impairments, disabilities or handicaps (Badley 1993; Wood 1980). The consequences are seen in terms of impairment, disability and handicap. *Impairment* is concerned with abnormalities in the structure or functioning of the body, *disability* with the performance of activities and *handicap* with the broader social and psychological consequences of living with impairment and disability. This classification has been applied to the understanding of aphasia (Jordan and Kaiser 1996). It is important to make clear that the relationship between these concepts is not inflexible. The severity of the impairment, for example, is not necessarily related to the severity of the disability or handicap that results. Locker (1997) describes two studies looking at people with multiple sclerosis and chronic respiratory disease which found that the severity of the condition did not predict the severity of the disability. Although there have been some criticisms of the use of the word 'handicap' (that is, it implies criticism of people and is arguably pejorative), in general the distinctions are useful and in clinical use. They serve to make our understanding of the individual's predicament more insightful. It is from this basis that our interest in the individual's interpretation of his or her situation has been explored.

The personal experience of chronic illness

Since there has been recognition of the qualitative approach to psychological research, there has been a developing literature on the personal perception of the individual. That is, particularly in cases of chronic illness, individuals come to form an understanding of their condition which allows them to *make sense of it*. In chronic conditions (such as aphasia) the individual makes an interpretation of the condition (for example, 'I can no longer rely on my speaking capacity') which is then tested out in many situations over a long period of time. As Bury (1991) states, 'in responding to chronic illness individuals constantly test the meanings attached to their altered situation against the reality of everyday experience'. The individual experiences regular comparisons between past self, present self and views of how he or she would wish to be. The aphasic speaker may, for example, have difficulty greeting some old friends and may hold a memory of how easily he would have done this before and how much he would like it to be easy again.

Recently there has been a huge increase in attention on the social effects of acquired communication impairment which has resulted in a far more sophisticated understanding of aphasic speakers in their social context (Jordan and Kaiser 1996; Parr et al. 1997). However, most of the literature on coping with chronic illness has disregarded the predicament of the aphasic speaker and assumed that the individual has language capacity which may aid adaptation. Gerhardt (1989), for example, has argued that language and communication are major ingredients in adaptation. The individual needs support in coping with a chronic disability. Having 'the ability to confide in others' (Bury 1991) may be denied to people with acquired communication impairment.

Bury (1991) has described the onset of chronic illness as a 'biographical disruption'. The notion behind this concept is that as well as the condition itself the context in which the illness occurs and the meaning it has for the individual all contribute to the capacity of the individual to cope. Bury distinguishes two types of meaning: first that which lies in its consequences for the individual. This is the immediate effects of the condition, including aspects of the medical regime or treatment procedures and how they disrupt everyday functioning. Second, is that relating to the social connotations or imagery associated with a condition. Thus, stereotyping and prejudice may affect the individual's coping strategy. For example, does the condition have a negative social presentation? People with stuttering difficulties are frequently perceived as being nervous. Of course, they may be nervous about a particular communicative event, but there is no evidence to suggest they are of a specifically nervous disposition. The 'does he take sugar' issue about people with obvious handicaps has relevance here. It is arguably more difficult to come to terms with a chronic disability if patients are aware that the social perception of them will change.

Various themes have been extrapolated in relation to the experience of chronic illness and Locker (1997) reports on these.

Uncertainty becomes part of experiencing a chronic condition. This may occur at the beginning of symptoms and relate to the individual's search for a diagnosis, and continue through to uncertainty about how to cope with later stages of an illness. The course and outcome of an illness is full of uncertainty, which means that planning in both the short and long term is affected. Family relationships (as previously discussed) can be affected by a chronic illness. Roles may change as an adaptation to the condition. The person with the condition may not enjoy relinquishing roles or may feel too much of a burden. Withdrawal by the family from society may occur as the result of the problems experienced.

Managing the medical regime may have a devastating effect upon the individual's life and family relationships. Many examples are quoted in the literature, such as coping with dialysis for kidney failure and the disruption to everyday life this may cause. Charmaz (1993) discusses a man who had defined the dialysis machine as an enemy and tried to make a friend or ally of the new kidney transplant that his body then began to reject. To this man the new kidney meant a much preferred identity and a route to a normal life as a student. To find that his body was rejecting it physically in spite of his mind wanting it psychologically was a source of great tension and distress.

Becoming aware of death is another aspect to the predicament of the chronically ill. Whatever the condition, the individual may experience a dilemma when the realisation takes place that death could occur. In a study on chronically ill men, Charmaz noted that awakening to death comes as a tremendous shock when an individual sees himself as too young to die, defines himself as exceptionally healthy or has had no earlier episodes heralding symptoms. Charmaz describes it as a 'sense of betrayal by their bodies' (p. 270) evoking anger, self-pity and envy of the healthy.

The personal understanding of the aphasic speaker has been well explored in the last decade. Frequently, aphasic people are excluded from studies of stroke because of the communication deficit, but Parr et al. (1997) were able to interview 50 aphasic speakers in order to develop important themes about the personal meaning of being aphasic. Many aspects to being aphasic are described, including perceptions of work, leisure, family and how all of this is affected by being aphasic. As the authors note, 'Language is the currency of relationships. It is used to invite, to suggest, to question, to advise, to argue, to reprimand, to bargain, to joke and to reassure' (p. 44). Thus all facets of life are affected and the aphasic speaker is in a particularly difficult situation being without the language skills to describe the experience. However, as Parr et al. revealed, being aphasic is not a barrier to communicating experience. One of the respondents interviewed described the experience as 'like opening doors and there's nothing in there' (p. 105).

Brumfitt (unpublished 1997) found that two aphasic speakers were able to reflect on their selfhood. Both were able to recognise the complexity of their situation and the feelings associated with it. As Client A said: 'Words are the gateway of do I say this or that or the other.'

How can an understanding of health psychology be applied in the speech and language therapy context?

In any type of speech and language therapy intervention we have to take into account the individual's understanding of the therapy process and the health care involved. So far the relationship of this to the outcome of speech and language therapy has been underdeveloped, but many applications from existing clinical psychology settings can be made. For example, many speech and language therapy interventions involve the individual in some form of behavioural change. This may particularly rely on self-directed behavioural change; that is the therapist requires the client or patient to take some responsibility for bringing about the change. In health contexts this can refer to stopping a behaviour which may lead to poor health, such as stopping smoking or changing poor eating habits. In speech and language therapy the analogy can be made with changing speech behaviours which disrupt the communicative process. Examples of this may be changing from being a stuttering speaker to being a fluent speaker, changing from being a speaker who abuses his or her voice to a speaker who has good vocal attack. Mahoney and Arnkoff (1979) describe the behaviours required in order to bring about behavioural change and these are described here with changing stuttering behaviour used as an example.

Self-monitoring

The individual needs to have a good understanding of actual behaviours before attempting to change them. Initially, the individual needs to keep records of the behaviour in the form of a diary, recording the number of behavioural events which are related to the piece of behaviour which may need to be changed and so on. The stuttering client would need to keep a record of the number of stuttering events in one day and in one week, with specific records of the conversational context in which this took place.

Goal specification

The therapist and client need to spend time on setting goals that are realistic and relevant for the client's problem. The self-monitoring records can be used as an aid here to develop a procedure that is embedded in the client's social context. For example, an unrealistic goal would be for a client with a substantial stuttering problem to aim to give a speech in public after a few short sessions of therapy and before useful fluency techniques had been learnt. A more realistic goal would include short-term goals for achieving fluency in controlled reading situations before moving on to controlled speaking situations. Long-term goals would include achieving an acceptable level of fluency within the social context of that individual.

Stimulus control

Procedures which affect the behaviour need to be taken into account. In the case of trying to reduce weight, for example, the physical environment could be controlled in order to help achieve more effective change. The individual would be encouraged to avoid eating in restaurants where there was a lot of temptation. In the case of the stuttering client the environment could be controlled by practice tasks with a controlled number and type of conversational partners. Included in this would be efforts to control internal factors too, such as self-defeating thoughts or beliefs like 'It's impossible to lead a normal life if I stop eating cakes' or 'It's impossible to lead a normal life if I keep having to control my fluency levels'. The client could be encouraged to make conscious efforts to make a decision to do something enjoyable every day in order to focus attention on positive feelings and beliefs.

Self-reinforcement

The principle here is that the individual must not find anything rewarding in the behaviour which is requiring change. Thus in the case of weight reduction, one of the difficulties is helping the individual find another 'rewarding' taste to substitute for the loss of saltiness in chips which has made the overweight person return to eating them regularly. In the stuttering speaker, any hidden rewards in stuttering must be identified. A relatively common example of this is the stutterer relying on others to make conversation so that avoidance of responsibility in conversational interaction becomes rewarding and thus impedes progress.

Social support

Implicit in behavioural change is the need for social support, otherwise individuals will be unable to make profound changes in their lifestyle. The importance of social support is well known in communication impairment and change.

Self-efficacy in the health context

This has relevance here in the same way as it does in the purely psychological context. Bandura (1977) established self-efficacy theory as a means of accounting for personal behaviour and how change may be generated. The core of the theory lies in the premise that the initiation and maintenance of behaviours are determined by:

a outcome values (the importance of certain outcomes, consequences or goals
b outcome expectancy (expectations concerning the effectiveness of certain behavioural means in producing those outcomes

c self-efficacy expectancy (judgements and expectations concerning behavioural skills and capabilities and the likelihood of being able successfully to implement the selected courses of action).

Clearly, this theory has relevance to the delivery of any sort of therapeutic procedure where behavioural change is an aim. The outcome of the therapy is dependent on the individual's self-belief about achieving mastery of the new behaviour.

Low self-efficacy expectancies may lead individuals to give up or stop trying to be effective in their lives. However, Maddux (1991) points out that these expectancies (whether high or low) are not necessarily diagnostic. Having a low self-efficacy does not imply psychological dysfunction. It does give an indication of subjective distress and how it will affect the individual's coping ability.

Research in this area has been applied to the phobic problem. Self-efficacy expectancies have been found to be reliable predictors of the phobic individual's ability to approach the feared stimuli. It has been demonstrated in phobias of snakes and spiders, heights, driving and the dark. That is, those who have strong belief about being able to undertake the behavioural programme required to rid them of a phobia are more likely to succeed than those who are unsure about their ability to do so.

In the self-efficacy model, depression is predicted under conditions of high outcome value, high outcome expectancy and low self-efficacy expectancy. That is, the individual who views something as extremely important, with associated high rewards, but believes him or herself to be unable to achieve the necessary behaviours to obtain the desired outcome, may be vulnerable to depression. A clinical example of this might be the adult with a stuttering problem who is required to speak in public in a work context. This individual views this event as critically important, and something which may enhance his career. However, he views the use of slowed speech technique as not necessarily reliable and believes his capacity for speaking in public as unpredictable and poor. The individual with beliefs like this will be vulnerable to depression and then find it even more difficult to cope with the communication problem. Maddux recommends an assessment of self-efficacy before any sort of treatment commences that can then be used as a baseline and also help a therapist target any competency beliefs that might be areas of concern. Many psychotherapeutic approaches aim to help the individual attain a sense of personal mastery whatever the presenting condition. Interestingly, this has never been fully explored in the speech and language therapy context, yet the relevance of this is obvious.

In terms of a working model of self-efficacy, there are three major cognitions which operate and can be assessed. These are referred to by Connor and Norman (1996) and provide a clear approach to increasing understanding about the way the individual is motivated to respond to therapeutic intervention (see Figure 5.2).

Risk perception
My risk of losing my voice is

Very low   *Low*   *High*   *Very high*

Outcome expectancy
If I stopped shouting in the classroom, then it would reduce my risk of losing my voice.

Not all true   *Barely true*   *Somewhat true*   *Very true*

Perceived self-efficacy
I am certain that I can stop shouting even when the children in my class misbehave.

Not at all true   *Barely true*   *Somewhat true*   *Very true*

Figure 5.2. Sample model

The key factor in the example given in Figure 5.2 is that by answering merely three single questions, it would be possible to gain an understanding of the likely success of an intervention for voice abuse. The answers here would be able to indicate very quickly what cognitive factors were influencing a response to intervention. Connor and Norman (1996) recommend that it is also essential to identify the individual's motivation to comply with intervention and suggest the use of a 'contemplation ladder' (Biener and Abrans 1991). A modified version of this is shown in Figure 5.3.

Each rung on this ladder represents where various people are in their thinking about voice use. Circle the number that indicates where you are now.

10 Taking action to stop shouting and other aspects of vocal abuse

9

8 Starting to think about how to change my voice use

7

6

5 Think I should use a soft attack to voice but still not quite ready

4

3 Think I need to do something about my voice

2

1

0 Not thought about my voice use

Figure 5.3. A contemplation ladder

Clearly, just by implementing these simple tasks the therapeutic procedure could be much improved and an increased understanding of selection of clients for intervention would be an implicit gain from the approach.

Enhancing the communicative context for the elderly person: health care applications

There are other ways of changing behaviour in a health care context which are relevant here. Although elderly people are more likely to suffer illness, changes also occur for the person who grows old without specific pathology. Elderly people have to make natural adjustments to increasing old age and can suffer from many aspects of ageing which affect their communicative competence. As individuals grow older they experience physical changes (such as deterioration in hearing and vision), cognitive changes and psychosocial changes. The capacity for communication continues to be critical for maintaining social and family relationships and for keeping control over the quality of life and everyday functioning.

As Lubinski and Welland (1997, p. 108) state: 'the environment that enhances communication can be one of the most powerful tools for enabling elders to live maximally independent, secure and fulfilling lives'. They suggest that various aspects of the environment can be modified to help. First, the acoustic environment is a source of difficulty if the individual has hearing difficulties. Recommendations include enhancing hearing abilities with assistive devices such as the variety of personal hearing aids available, telephone support devices, television and radio devices and alerting aids. Second, partners can learn to use communication enhancing strategies such as maintaining face-to-face communication, gaining the person's attention before beginning a conversation, rephrasing and repeating important information and making clear introductions or shifts in topic during conversations. In addition, attempts should be made to ensure that background noise is limited and making sure that a conversation is attempted only when background noise has been controlled.

The visual environment is another factor in the elderly person's communicative problem. Non-verbal information is a critical part of the way in which we understand what is being said to us. We rely on non-verbal behaviours to provide the impact of the message and it can account for a great part of the emotional effect of what the speaker is trying to convey. Lubinski and Welland recommend an approach which facilitates the individual's ability to perceive non-verbal cues. First, and most obviously, they recommend that great care is given to providing the individual with the necessary visual support devices. Second, that visual information is modified to facilitate accurate perception – this includes ensuring that important visual information is placed at eye level, such as clocks, calendars and noticeboards. Also use of colour can be incorporated into the environment, such as using colour contrasts rather than coordinates. Health care assistants, if colour coded, can be organised so that contrasting colours are used. Improving the actual physical environment is also essential. Illumination and lighting methods are extremely important – elderly people require two or three times as much illumination but are also very sensitive to direct and indirect glare. Appropriate lighting of halls, steps and entrances is crucial. Placement of furniture can be manipulated to facilitate ease of movement and accessibility. Arrangement of furniture is necessary to ensure that conversation can take place more easily with partners sitting opposite one another at comfortable eye-level viewing range. There is some evidence to show that an elderly person's depth perception changes with age. In particular, distinguishing an object on a patterned background can be more problematic with advanced age and care must taken in relation to floor surfaces.

As well as ensuring a good environment, the effectiveness of communication is dependent on the quality of the conversational interaction. Erber (1994) discusses the deterioration of communication in the ageing person if the environment is not sufficiently enhanced or support or advice offered to potential partners. This is particularly so in residential settings where the quality of communication is frequently cited as poor. Health care workers, family and friends may need guidance in how to communicate with an elderly resident even in the absence of pathological communication disorder. There is much variation between residential homes for the elderly, but many do recognise the importance of providing the correct physical environment. Le Dorze et al. (1994) investigated the types of communicative interaction which took place within an institutionalised setting with different groups of care givers (nurses, orderlies, professionals and volunteers) to establish the nature of the interaction for residents with no communication handicap, aphasic speakers and residents with dementia. Following qualitative analysis of interviews with these care givers the results showed that communication in daily life situations varied little between the different groups. However, residents with communication impairment are perceived to be less involved in communicative acts than residents with no communication impairment.

Erber takes the view that many limit opportunities for conversation merely by unwritten codes of behaviour within that setting, and discusses the limits placed on the elderly if there are no opportunities for talking with the opposite sex, talking late at night, and even the self-regulatory behaviour of elderly people in their tendency to talk only with a limited number of people, excluding anybody who is perceived as 'different'. Erber recommends that professional intervention should be provided for elderly institutionalised people taking into account the following criteria.

The person's ability to perceive and comprehend language

The person's capacity for conversational fluency: recurring need for conversational repair may lead to frustration, lowered self-esteem and subsequent avoidance of communication

The importance of communicative success or failure to the individual

The person's level of cognitive functioning: a person with poor retention may require more frequent interaction, because the effects of social activity may quickly diminish

The amount of daily social interaction with other residents or staff or visitors

The topic and context of regular interaction (complexity and interest to the client)

The amount of other communicative contact, e.g. watching television, talking to a pet

The individual's personality type, cultural background, former communication patterns, habits and current social needs. (1994, p. 272)

As Maxim and Bryan (1994) point out, the way the elderly person responds to intervention may be different to the younger age group and as with the criteria listed above this always needs to be acknowledged. Although age is not the absolute factor in potential for recovery, what does seem to be critical is the presence of other health-related factors and these, as Maxim and Bryan indicate, are much more likely to be seen in the older person.Thus, even if the individual does not have specific pathological impairments, they will be suffering from health problems which may affect their motivation and capacity for communication.

Because the elderly person has to come into contact with health care professionals there has been some research to look at the effectiveness of communication between the elderly and the professional. Lubinski and Welland (1997) report a project which investigated the nature of miscommunications between elderly people and nurses during 20 admission interviews to general medical surgical wards in a US hospital. Results showed that there were six sources of miscommunication between nurse interviewers and elders: the acoustic background; unclear phonology or syntax of the nurse resulting in ambiguous or vague questions; the nurse's use of medical terminology; unclear or incomplete communication from the elderly person to the nurse which was ignored; difficulty by either party in understanding the communicative intent; and statements made by the nurses which were not believed by the elderly people. This study alerts us to the issues involved in communicating with the elderly as a care group and the potential role the speech and language therapist can play in educating the health professional about good and effective communicative styles with different care groups.

Summary

Many of the aspects of health psychology discussed here have not yet been transferred to the speech and language therapy context; for example, we do not use health belief models routinely when evaluating a client or parental response to advice. We overlook issues to do with compliance, yet clearly our role with both clients and relatives requires it. One of the most positive ways we have developed our knowledge base is by applying the social model of understanding of health to many of our client groups. The work on chronic illness and disability is directly relevant to our work with many of the acquired conditions. The recent literature in aphasiology demonstrates this (Jordan and Kaiser 1996; Parr et al. 1997). Recognising that people with communication impairments need to feel empowered in their own social contexts is a huge shift in the way we approach our clients. Using locus of control scales to evaluate the beliefs of the individual would greatly increase our clinical sensitivity to factors yet unexplored in response to speech and language therapy. Recognising that the beliefs and values an individual has before entering therapy may be critical to outcome is one way in which the process of therapy could be enhanced.

Exercise

The client you are working with has a voice problem associated with working in a smoky atmosphere and having hobbies which involve both shouting and speaking in public (football matches and amateur dramatics). The client is a 45-year-old man who smokes and drinks and is overweight. He lives in a small town and commutes daily by car to his place of work in a city 20 miles away.

Are this man's health beliefs relevant in this situation? If they are, how would you investigate this?

Recommended reading

Banyard P (1996) Applying Psychology to Health. London: Hodder and Stoughton.
Bennet P, Murphy S (1997) Psychology and Health Promotion. Buckingham: Open University Press.
Sarno MT (1997) Quality of life in aphasia in the first post stroke year. Aphasiology 11(7): 665–79.

Conclusion

Throughout the chapters of this book we have seen the different ways in which an individual with a communication handicap may be influenced by various social and health factors. We began by looking at the individual's sense of self and identity and how this can be affected by handicap. Through the other chapters we moved towards an understanding of the ways psychology in a health context can be influential. The book began with the individual context but became more expansive taking in the wider context of the family, psychological stages in life and how we function in ill health.

The material therefore gives us a wider perspective on the person with a speech and language impairment. On meeting with a client we see a person with an individual identity but set in a family structure and influenced by other factors that arise out of growing older and experiencing good or bad health. We cannot therefore view the dysphasic speaker as nothing but a dysphasic speaker or a child with a phonological impairment as nothing but a child with that problem. Each client who we meet comes with a multidimensional set of views and experiences and we need to incorporate those into our professional perception of them. We disregard them at our peril.

Chapter 1 on the self and identity showed that self-understanding may be critical in a therapeutic programme. It was possible to demonstrate ways in which the self can be described and measured and the way in which this understanding can be applied to the communicative disability context. In theory, measurement of self could be used in a baseline speech and language therapy assessment and contribute to the wider therapeutic understanding. If this became an accepted part of service delivery then there would also be a much greater scope for developing more scales to measure self in people with communication disability. As described in this chapter, there are special problems with measuring self if there is language impairment; a greater awareness and debate of this would ensure the development of further research.

Chapter 2, looking at attitudes, draws attention to the importance of understanding the role of attitudes in the health care context. There is already some application of the work on attitudes towards disability and the attitudes of people with disabilities to the special client groups of the communicatively disabled. Much of this work started with the stuttering syndrome but it has now been applied to the people with acquired impairments and those with congenital communication impairments too. For the future we need to identify the attitudes which may offer a profile of other client groups with communication impairments. We need to know whether attitude towards the communication disability can influence therapeutic outcome and also whether attitude towards a therapeutic programme makes any substantial difference.

Life transitions clearly affect all of us and so do life events. In Chapter 3 we can explore the ways in which we share some of the same experiences as our clients. Sometimes we have had the same experiences as our clients, such as moving from childhood to adolescence and then to adulthood and middle age, and on other occasions the experience is way beyond anything we may experience ourselves. But we also need to keep in mind disrupted transition or delayed transition, which may occur because of the variety of aetiologies our clients may experience.

Understanding the ways families function is a core part of the speech and language therapist's work. The family has a powerful influence on the child or adult with a communication impairment. The therapist needs the support of the family in order to make the best use of therapy, and a supportive family can facilitate more developments than a child or adult in isolation practising communication tasks. Families of children with handicap, for example, can be critical in helping to provide an additional source of training if a remedial programme is created. In addition, however, the therapist has to recognise that the source of distress or difficulty with coping may lie within the family context for many clients who have communication impairments. A therapist has to be knowledgeable about what can go wrong in a family; this may be quite independent of the communication impairment and many of our clients have to function within family settings which are far from ideal. Thus, knowing about the family is critical to what clinical decisions a therapist may take. A child from a family with dysfunction may be managed in an entirely different way to a child from a stable family. As health professionals, speech and language therapists deal with these issues on a daily basis, but we can, through further research, learn to understand more clearly those factors in the family context that may have direct influences upon the progress of treatment procedures.

The contribution of psychology to the understanding of health matters has grown considerably in the last decade. Matters that were previously regarded as exclusively medical now have a psychological interpetation put upon them. We must note how much this has helped the patient or client. All illnesses have psychological aspects and the recognised status of this within a health context has led all professionals to a more sophisticated understanding of medical conditions. It is this interaction between the people with the communication impairment and their health beliefs and attitudes that will benefit from the further research by speech and language therapists. Health psychology research into major illnesses, such as cancer and diabetes and patients' reactions and coping strategies has already been done. We can hope that more research can be developed for those with communication impairments. The final chapter has presented many of the areas where we could apply this research directly to speech and language therapy, but we want to be able to describe this more accurately in relation to our own client groups. The more we are able to understand these factors the better we will be able to develop programmes of therapy which can create a better quality of life.

In the next millenium, there is hope that there will be a drawing together of social and health psychology with speech and language therapy practice. Evidence for our practice is needed from a wide variety of sources and in social and health psychology we have a wide and an exciting field on which to draw.

References

Alder B (1995) Psychology of Health. Luxemberg: Harwood Academic Publishers.

Altschuler J (1997) Working with Chronic Illness. London: Macmillan.

Anderson R (1992) The Aftermath of Stroke. Cambridge: Cambridge University Press.

Anderson R, Bury M (1988) Living with Chronic Illness: The Experience of Patients and Their Families. London: Unwin Hyman.

Andrews G, Cutler J (1974) Stuttering therapy: the relation between changes in symptom level and attitudes. Journal of Speech and Hearing Disorders 39: 312–19.

Antonius K, Beukelman D, Reid R (1996) Communicative disablity of Parkinson's disease – percpetions of dysarthric speakers and their primary communication partners. In Robin D, Yorkston K, Beukelman D (eds) Disorders of Motor Speech Assessment and Treatment and Clinical Characterisation. New York: Paul Brookes Publishing Company.

Badeley A (1993) Your Memory: A Users Guide, 2nd edn. Harmondsworth: Penguin.

Badley E (1993) An introduction to the concepts and classifications of the international classification of impairments, disabilities and handicaps. Disabil. Rehab. 15 161–78.

Bandura A (1977) Social Learning Theory. Englewood Cliffs, NJ: Prentice Hall.

Banford F (1989) in Meadow R (ed) ABC of child abuse. London. British Medical Journal.

Banyard P (1996) Applying Psychology to Health. London: Hodder and Stoughton.

Barratt H, Jones D (1996) The inner life of children with moderate learning disabilities. In Varma VP (ed.) The Inner Life of Children with Special Needs. London: Whurr.

Bartlett FC (1932) Remembering: An Experimental and Social Study. Cambridge: Cambridge University Press.

Bartlett LB, Limsila P (1992) Severe deprivation in childhood: a case report from Thailand. British Journal of Psychiatry 161: 412–14.

Baum A, Gatchel R, Krantz L (1997) An Introduction to Health Psychology. New York: McGraw Hill.

Baumeister RF (1995) Self and Identity: An Introduction. In Tesser A (ed.) Advanced Social Psychology. New York: McGraw Hill.

Baumrind D (1973) The development of instrumental competence through socialisation. In Pick AD (ed.) Minnesota Symposia on Child Psychology, Vol. 7. Minneapolis, MN: University of Minnesota Press.

Bellaby P (1993) The world of the closed head injured. In Radley A (ed.) Worlds of Illness. New York: Tavistock-Routledge.

Bennet P, Murphy S (1997) Psychology and Health Promotion. Buckingham: Open University Press.

Biener L, Abrams DB (1991) The contemplation ladder: validation of a measure of readiness to consider smoking cessation. Health Psychology 10, 360–5.

Blane D (1997) Health professions. In Scrambler G (ed) Sociology as Applied to Medicine. London: WB Saunders.

Blaskovich J, Tomaka J (1991) Measures of Self Esteem. Measure of Personality and Social Psychological Attitudes: Academic Press.

Block JR, Yuker HE (1979) Attitudes towards disability are the key. Rehabilitation Digest 10: 2–3.

Bohannon P (1971) Divorce and After: An analysis of the emotional and social problems of divorce. Garden City, NY: Anchor.

Borland M (1976) Violence in the Family. New York: Manchester University Press.

Boisclair-Papillon R (1983) The family of the person with aphasia. In Lafond D, DeGiovanni R, Joanette Y. Ponzio J, Taylor Sarno M, (eds) Living With Aphasia. San Diego California: Singular Publishing Group.

Brumfitt SM (1985) The use of repertory grids with aphasic people. In Beail N (ed.) Repertory Grid technique and Personal Constructs. London: Croom Helm.

Brumfitt SM, Clarke PRF (1983) An application of psychotherapeutic techniques to the management of aphasia. In Code C, Muller D (eds) Aphasia Therapy. London: Edward Arnold.

Brumfitt SM, Sheeran P (1997) An evaluation of short-term group therapy for people with aphasia. Disability and Rehabilitation 19(6): 221–31.

Brumfitt SM (1997) (unpublished) PhD thesis. The personal meaning of aphasia.

Brumfitt SM, Sheeran P (1999) VASES: The Visual Analogue Self-Esteem Scale. Bicester: Winslow Press.

Brumfitt SM, Atkinson J, Greated C (1994) The carer's response to written information about acquired communication problems. Aphasiology (19(6) 221–31.

Brutten GJ, Dunham S (1989) The communication attitude test: a normative study of grade school children. Journal of Fluency Disorders 414: 371–7.

Burns RB (1979) The Self Concept. London: Longman.

Bury M (1991) The sociology of chronic illness: a review of research and prospects. Sociology of Health and Illness 13: 451-68.

Butler JM, Haigh GV (1954) Changes in the relation between self concept and ideal self concept consequent upon client centred counselling. In Burns RB (ed. (1979) The Self Concept. London: Longman.

Button E (1987) Construing people or weight? An eating disorders group. In Neimayer RA, Meimayer GJ (eds) Personal Construct Therapy Casebook. New York: Springer.

Button E (1990) Rigidity of construing of self and significant others and psychological disorder. British Journal of Medical Psychology 63: 345–54.

Byrne B (1996) Measuring the Self-concept Across the Life Span. Washington DC: American Psychological Association.

Carr A, Personal constructs of aphasic speakers and right hemisphere damaged speakers. Unpublished MPhil.

Charmaz K (1983) The grounded theory method.: an explication and interpetation. In Emerson RM (ed) Contemporary Field Research. Boston MA: Little Brown.

Charmaz L (1995) The body, identity and self: adapting to impairment. The Sociological Quarterly 36(4): 657–680.

Cohen LH (1988) Life Events and Psychological Functioning. London: Sage.

Coleman P (1993) Psychological aging. In Bond S, Coleman P, Pearce S (eds) Aging in Society. London: Sage.

Connor M, Norman P (1996 (eds) Predicting Health Behaviour. Buckingham: Open University Press.

Conti Ramsden G, Dykins SJ (1991) Mother–child interactions with language impaired children and their siblings. British Journal of Disorders of Communication 26(3): 337–55.

Dalton P (ed) (1983) Approaches to the Treatment of Stuttering. London: Croom Helm.

Dalton P (1994) Counselling People with Communication Problems. London: Sage.

Dalton P, Hardcastle B (1977) Disorders of Fluency. London: Arnold.

Daly DA (1992) Helping the clutterer: therapy considerations. In Myers FL, St Louis KO (eds) Cluttering: A Clinical Perspective. Kibworth: Far Communications.

Darvill G (1983) Rehabilitation – not just voice. In Edels Y (ed.) Laryngectomy: diagnosis to rehabilitation. London: Croom Helm.

DeNil LF, Brutten G, Claeys M (1986) Stutterers and non-stutterers – a normative investigation on children's speech associated attitudes. Paper given at the ASHA convention, Washington.

DeNil LF, Kroll RM (1995) The relationship between locus of control and long term stuttering treatment outcome in adult stutterers. Journal of Fluency Disorders 29: 79–83.

Department of Health (1993) Health of the Nation Key Handbook: Coronary Heart Disease and Stroke. London. DoH.

Duck S (1986) Human Relationships. London: Sage.

Ebrahim S, Baer D, Nouri F (1987) Affective illness after stroke. British Journal of Psychiatry 151: 56–7.

Ellis DA, Hopkin JM, Leitch AG, Croften J (1979) Doctors' orders: controlled trial of supplementary written information for patients. British Medical Journal (1) 456.

Emler N (1993) The young person's relationship to the institutional order. In Jackson S, Rodriguez-Tome (eds) Adolescence and its Social Worlds. Hove: Lawrence Erlbaum.

Epting FR (1984) Personal Construct Counselling and Psychotherapy. New York: Wiley.

Erber NP (1994) Conversation as therapy for older adults in residential care: the case for intervention. European Journal of Disorders of Communication 29(3): 269–79.

Erikson E (1965) Childhood and Society. Harmondsworth: Penguin/Hogarth Press.

Erikson EH (1980) Identity and the Life Cycle – A Reissue. New York: Norton.

Erikson RL (1969) Assessing communication attitudes among stutterers. JSHR 12: 711–214.

Festinger L (1954) A theory of social comparison processes. Human Relations 7: 117–40.

Festinger L (1957) A Theory of Cognitive Dissonance. Evanston IL: Row Peterson.

Festinger L (1964) Conflict, Decision and Dissonance. Stanford CA: Stanford University Press.

Field T (1978) Interaction behaviours of primary versus secondary caretaker fathers. Developmental Psychology 14: 183–4.

Fiske S, Taylor SE (1992) Social Cognition, 2nd edn. New York: McGraw-Hill.

Flavell JH, Miller IH, Miller SA (1993) Cognitive Development, 3rd edn. Englewood Cliffs NJ: Prentice Hall.

Flesch R (1948) A new readability yardstick. Journal of Applied Psychology 32: 221–33.

Fogarty TF (1976) System concepts and the dimension of self. In PJ Guerin (ed.) Family Therapy, Theory and Practice. New York: Gardner.

Foon AE (1987) Review: locus of control as a predictor of outcome of psychotherapy. British Journal of Medical Psychology 60: 99–107.

Fox N, Sobel A, Calkins S, Cole P (1996) Inhibited children talk about themselves: self reflection on personality development and change in 7-year-olds. In Lewis M, Wolan Sullivan, M (eds) Emotional Development in Atypical Children. Hove: Lawrence Erlbaum.

Fransella F (1972) Personal Change and Reconstruction. New York: Academic Press.

Fransella F, Adams B (1966) An illustration of the use of repertory grid technique in a clinical setting. British Journal of Social Clinical Psychology 5: 51–63.

Fry E (1987) Disabled People and the 1987 General Election. London: Spastics Society.

Garcia Torres B (1990) Development of self-descriptions in the context of play: a longitudinal study. In Oppenheimer L (ed.) The Self Concept. New York: Springer.

Garrett B (1992) Gerontology and communication disorders: a model for training clincians. Educational Gerontology 18(3): 231–42

Gerhardt U (1989) Ideas about illness: an intellectual and political history of medical sociology. London: Macmillan.

Gillham B (1994) Child Physical Abuse. London: Cassell.

Glozman ZM, Tsyganok AA (1982) Some aspects of personality change in aphasia. Soviet Neurology and Psychiatry 16: 15–26.

Gordon A (1977) Thinking with restricted language a personal construct investigation of prelingually profoundly deaf apprentices. British Journal of Psychology 68: 253–5.

Gregory HH (1979) Controversies About Stuttering Therapy. Baltimore MD: University Park Press.

Gregory S, Bishop J, Sheldon L (1995) Deaf Young People and Their Families. Cambridge: Cambridge University Press.

Groze V and Ileana D (1996) Successful Adoptive Families: A Longitudinal Study of Special Needs Adoption. New York: Praeder.

Hattie, J. (1992) Self Concept. Hove: Lawrence Erlbaum.

Hayhow R, Levy C (1989) Working with Stuttering. Bicester: Winslow Press.

Health and Personal Social Services Statistics for England (1997) London: The Stationery Office.

Herrman M, Wallesch CW (1989) Psychosocial changes and psychosocial adjustment in aphasia in a MAUT study with the Code Muller Scale of Psychosocial adjustment. Aphasiology 4: 527–38.

Hillier S, Scambler G (1997) Women as patients and providers. In Scambler G (ed.) Sociology as Applied to Medicine. London: WB Saunders.

Hodgins E (1968) Episode: Report on the Accident Inside My Skull. New York: Atheneum.

Hoen B, Thelander M, Worsley J (1997) Improvement in psychological well-being of people with aphasia and their families: evaluation of a community-based programme. Aphasiology 11(7): 681–91.

Holmes TH, Rahe RH (1967) The social readjustment rating scale. Journal of Psychosomatic Research 11: 213–18.

Horrocks J, Jackson D (1972) Self and Role. Boston MA: Houghton and Mifflin.

Horsley IA, Fitzgibbon CT (1987) Stuttering children: an investigation of a stereotype. British Journal of Disorders of Communication 22(1): 19–37.

Howitt D, Billig M, Cramer D, Edwar S, Kniveton B, Potter J, Radley A (1992) Social Psychology: Conflicts and Continuities. Buckingham: Open University Press.

Jackson S (1990) A self characterisation; development and deviance in adolescent construing. In Winter D (1992) Personal Construct Theory in Clinical Practice. London: Routledge.

Jackson S, Bannister D (1985) Growing into self. In Bannister D (ed.) Issues and Approaches in Personal Construct Theory. London: Academic Press.

James S, Brumfitt SM, Cudd P (in press) Communicating by telephone: views of a group of people with stuttering impairment. Journal of Fluency Disorders.

James W (1890) Principles of Psychology. New York: Holt.

Joanette Y, Lafond D, Lecours AR (1993) The person and aphasia. In Lafond D,

Degiovani R, Joanette Y, Ponzio J, Taylor Sarno M (1993) Living with Aphasia. San Diego: California: Singular Publishing Group.

Jones CJ (1985) Analysis of the self concepts of handicapped students. Remedial and Special Education 6(5): 32–6.

Jordan L, Kaiser W (1996) Aphasia – a Social Approach. London: Chapman & Hall.

Kalinowski JS, Lerman JW, Watt J (1987) A preliminary examination of the perceptions of self and others in stutterers and non stutterers. Journal of Fluency Disorders 12: 317–331.

Kaplan C, Sallis J, Patterson T (1993) Health and Human Behaviour. New York: McGraw-Hill.

Kaplan RM, Bush JW (1982 Health related quality of life measurement for evaluation research and policy analysis. Health Psychology 1: 61–80.

Kasl SA, Cobb S (1966) Health behaviour illness behaviour and sick role behaviour. Archives of Environmental Health 12: 246–66.

Kelly G (1955) The Psychology of Personal Constructs. New York: Norton.

Kinsella G, Duffy, F (1979) Psychosocial readjustment in the spouses of aphasic patients. Scandinavian Journal of Rehabilitation Medicine 11

Koluchova J (1972) Severe deprivation in twins: a case study. In Clarke MA, Clarke ADB (ed.) Early Experience: Myth and Evidence. London: Open Books.

Koppitz EM (1968) Psychological Evaluation of Children's Human Figure Drawings. New York: Grune and Stratton.

Korsch BM, Gozzi EK, Francis V (1968) Gaps in doctor–patient communication. Paediatrics 42: 855–71.

Kuhn MH, McPartland TS (1954) An empirical investigation of self attitudes. American Sociological Review 19: 68–76.

Kunnen S (1990) Development of perceived competence in physically handicapped and non-handicapped children. In Oppenheimer AN (1966) Questionnaire Design and Attitude Meaurement. London; Heinemann.

Law J, Elias J (1996) Trouble Talking. London: Jessica Kingsley Publishers.

Le Dorze G, Julien M, Brassard C, Durocher J, Boivin G (1994) An analysis of the communication of adult residents of a long term hospital as perceived by their caregivers. European Journal of Disorders of Communication 29(3): 241–69.

Lefcourt HM (1976) Locus of Control: Current Trends in Theory and Research. Hillsdale NJ: Erlbaum.

Lewis C (1986) The role of the father in the human family. In Sluckin W, Herbert M (eds) Parental Behaviour. Oxford: Blackwell.

Ley P (1988) Communicating with Patients. New York: Croom Helm.

Ley P (1988) Memory for medical information. British Journal of Social and Clinical Psychology 18, 245–256.

Locke JL (1993) The Child's Path to Spoken Language. London: Harvard University Press.

Locker D (1997) Living with chronic illness. In Scambler G (ed.) Sociology as Applied to Medicine, 4th edn. London: WB Saunders.

Lorenzini R, Sassasoli S, Rocchi MT (1988) The construction of change in agoraphobia. In Fransella F, Thomas L (eds) Experimenting with Personal Construct Psychology. London: Routledge.

Lubinski R, Welland R (1997) Normal aging and environmental affects on communication. Seminars in Speech and Language 18(2): 107–26.

Luepnitz DA (1986) A comparison of maternal, paternal and joint custody: understanding the varieties of post-divorce family life. Journal of Divorce 9: 1–12.

Luzatti C, Verga R (1996) Reduplicative paramnesia for patients with preserved memory. In Halligan P, Marshal J (eds) Methods in Madness. Hove: Psychology Press.

Maddux JE (1991) Self efficacy. In Snyder CR, Forsyth DR (eds) Handbook of Social and Clinical Psychology. New York: Pergamon.

Malone RL (1969) Expressed attitudes of families of aphasics. Journal of Speech and Hearing Disorders 34: 146–51.

Mancuso JC, Handin KH (1980) Training parents to construe the child's construing. In Landfield AW, Leitner L (eds) Personal Construct Psychology: Psychotherapy and Personality. New York: Wiley.

Maxim J, Bryan K (1994) Language of the Elderly. London: Whurr.

McKay AP, McKenna PJ, Laws K (1996) Severe schizophrenia what is it like? In Halligan P, Marshal J (eds) Methods in Madness. Hove: Psychology Press.

McLaughlin, H (1969) Smog rating: a new readability formula. Journal of Reading 22: 639–46.

McMullan SJ, Fisher L (1992) Developmental progress of Romanian orphanage children in Canada. Canadian Psychology 33(2): 504.

McNeil MC, Polloway EA, Smith D (1984) Feral and isolated children: historical review and analysis. Education and Training of the Mentally Retarded, February: 70–9,

Meadow KP (1980) Deafness and Child Development. London: Edward Arnold.

Morris LA, Groft S (1982) Patient package inserts: a research perspective. In Melmon K (ed) Drug Therapeutic Concepts for Clinicians. New York: Elsevier.

Mulhall D (1978) Dysphasic stroke patients and the influence of their relatives. British Journal of Disorders of Communication 13: 127–34.

Murray Parkes C (1975) Bereavement. London: Pelican.

Myers FL, St Louis KO (1992) Cluttering: A Clinical Perspective. Kibworth: Far Communication.

Nelson Jones R (1986) Human Relationship Skills. London: Cassell.

Nelson Jones R (1991) The Theory and Practice of Counselling Psychology. London: Cassell.

Nicholls F, Varchevker A, Pring, T (1996) Working with people with aphasia and their families: an exploration of the use of family therapy techniques. Aphasiology 10 (8) 767–81.

Niemi M, Laaksonen R, Kotila M, Waltimo O (1988) Quality of life four years after stroke. Stroke 19(9): 1101–7.

Niven N (1994) Health Psychology. London: Churchill Livingstone.

Oliver M, Zarb G (1997) The politics of disability: a new approach. In Barton L, Oliver M (eds) Disability Studies. Leeds: The Disability Press.

Osgood CE, Suci GT, Tannenbaum PH (1957) The Measurement of Meaning. Urbana IL: University of Illinois.

Palmore E (1977) Facts on ageing: a short quiz. The Gerontologist 17: 315–20.

Parr S, Byng S, Gilpin S, Ireland C (1997) Talking About Aphasia. Buckingham: Open University Press.

Partridge C, Johnston M (1989) Perceived control over recovery from physical disability: measurement and prediction. British Journal of Clinical Psychology 28: 53–9.

Pelham BW, Swann WB (1989) From self conceptions to self worth: on the sources and structure of low self esteem. Journal of Personality and Social Psychology 57: 670–2.

Petty R (1995) Attitude change. In Tesser A (ed.) Advanced Social Psychology. New York: McGraw Hill.

Piaget J (1936/52) The Origin of Intelligence in the Child. London. Routledge and Kegan Paul.

Piers EV, Harris D (1984) Piers-Harris Children's Self Concept Scale. Revised manual. Los Angeles, CA: Western Psychology Services.

Pruyn JFA, DeJong PC, Bosman JW, Van Poppel MJ, Van Den Borne HW, Ryckman RM, De Meij K (1986) Psychosocial aspects of head and neck cancer – a review of the literature. Clinical Otolaryngology 11: 469–74.

Radford J (1990) Child Prodigies and Exceptional Early Achievers. New York: Harvester Wheatsheaf.

Reynell J (1969) A developmental approach to language disorders. British Journal of Disorders of Communication 4: 33–40.

Rinaldi W (1996) The inner life of youngsters with specific developmental language disorder. In Varma VP (ed.) The Inner Life of Children with Special Needs. London: Whurr.

Rogers CR, Dymond RF (1954) Psychotherapy and personality change. In Burns RB (ed.) The Self Concept. London: Longman.

Roid GH, Fitts WH (1994) Tennessee Self Concept Scale, Revised Manual. Los Angeles CA: Western Psychological Services.

Rollin W (1987) The Psychology of Communication Disorders in Individuals and their Families. Englewood Cliffs NJ: Prentice Hall.

Romano MD (1974) Family response to traumatic head injury. Scandinavian Journal of Rehabilitation Medicine 6: 1–4.

Ronis DL and Harely (1989) Health beliefs and breast self examination behaviours: analysis of linear structural relations. Psychology and Health Journal 259–285.

Ronis DL, Kaiser MK (1989) Correlates of breast self examination in a sample of college women analyes of linear structural relations. Journal of Applied Social Psychology (19) 1068–84.

Rosenberg M (1965) Society and the Adolescent Self Image. Princeton NJ: Princeton University Press.

Rosenberg GM (1979) Conceiving the Self. New York: Basic Books.

Rosenstock IM (1966) Why people use health services. Milbank Memorial Fund Quarterly 44: 94–127.

Roth HP, Caron HS, Ort RS, Berger DG, Merrill RS, Albee GW, Streeter GA (1962) Patients' belefs about peptic ulcer and its treatment. Annals of Internal Medicine 56: 72–80.

Rotter JB (1966a) Social Learning and Clinical Psychology. Englewood Cliffs NJ: Prentice Hall.

Rotter JB (1966b) Generalised expectancies for internal versus external control of reinforcement. Psychological Monographs 80.

Rubenstein SY (1970) Experimental procedures in abnormal psychology, Moscow. In Tyerman A, Humphrey M (1984) changes in self concept following severe head injury. International Journal of Rehabilitation Research 7(1): 11–23.

Rustin L (1991) Parents, Families and the Stuttering Child. Kibworth: Far Communication.

Rutter M (1967) Maternal Deprivation Reassessed. Harmondsworth: Penguin.

Sabat SR, Harre R (1992) The construction and reconstruction of self in Alhzeimer's disease. Aging and Society 12: 443–61.

Salmon P (1985) Living in Time. London: JM Dent and Sons.

Sarno MT (1997) Quality of life in aphasia in the first post stroke year. Aphasiology 11(7): 665–79.

Schaffer HR (1996) Social Development. Oxford: Blackwell.

Schwartz HD (1993) Adolescents who stutter. Journal of Fluency Disorders 20: 289–302.

Shadden B (1988) Perceptions of daily communicative interactions with older persons. In Shadden B (ed.) Communication Behaviour and Ageing. Baltimore MD: Williams Wilkins.

Shearer WM (1961) A theoretical consideration of the self concept and body image in stuttering therapy. Journal of American Speech and Hearing Association 3: 115–16.

Sheehan JG (1954) An integration of psychotherapy and speech therapy through a conflict theory of stuttering. Journal of Speech and Hearing Disorders XIX: 474–82.

Sheehan JG (1958) Conflict theory of stuttering. In Eisenson J (ed.) Stuttering: a Symposium. New York. Harper and Row.

Sheehan JG, Voas RB (1954) Tension patterns during stuttering in relation to conflict, anxiety binding and reinforcement. Speech Monographs XXI: 272–9.

Shontz F (1965) Reactions to crisis. Volta Review 65: 364–70.

Sillars A, Zietlow P (1993) Investigations of marital communication and lifespan development. In Coupland N, Nussbaum J (eds) Discourse and Lifespan Identity. Newbury Park CA: Sage.

Silverman EM (1980) Communication attitudes of women who stutter. Journal of Speech and Hearing Disorders XLV: 533–9.

Skuse D (1984) Extreme deprivation in early childhood. Theoretical Issues and a Comparative Review 25(4): 543–572.

Slater R (1984) Aging. In Gale A, Chapman AJ (1984) Psychology and Social Problems. New York: Wiley.

Smith P, Cowie H, Blades M. (1998) Understanding Children's Development. Oxford: Blackwell.

Snyder M, Miene P (1994) Stereotyping of the elderly: a functional approach. British Journal of Social Psychology 33: 63–82

Sokolov AN (1972) Inner Speech and Thought. New York: Plenum Press.

Speck P (1978) Loss and Grief in Medicine. London: Bailliere Tindall.

Spinelli E. (1989) The Interpreted World. London: Sage.

Stern RA, Arruda JE, Hooper CR, Wolfener GD, Morey CE (1997) Visual analogue mood scales to measure internal mood state in neurologically impaired patients; description and initial validity evidence. Aphasiology 11(1): 59–71.

Stevenson J, Richman N, Grahame P (1985) Behaviour problems and language abilities at 3 years and behaviour deviance at 8 years. Journal of Child Psychology and Psychiatry 26 (2): 215–30.

Stewart T (1982) The relationship of attitude and intentions to behave to the acquisiton of speech behaviour by stammerers. British Journal of Disorders of Communication 17: 3–13.

Stewart T (1987) Positive attitude to fluency a group therapy programme. In Levy C (ed.) Stuttering Therapies: Practical Approaches. London: Croom Helm.

Stewart T (1996) A further application of the Fishbein and Ajzen model to therapy with adult stammerers . European Journal of Disorders of Communication 31(4) 455–65.

Sutcliffe LM, Lincoln NB (1998) The assessment of depression in aphasic stroke patients: the development of the Stroke Aphasic Depression Questionnaire. Clinical Rehabilitation 12: 506–13.

Syder D (1998) Wanting to Talk. London: Whurr.

Tanner D, Gerstenberger D (1988) The grief response in neuropathologies of speech and language. Apahsiology 2: 79–84.

Tesser A (1995) Advances Social Psychology. New York: McGraw Hill.

Thomas D (1978) The Social Psychology of Childhood Disability. New York: Methuen.

Triplett N (1898) The dynamogenic factors in pacemaking and competition. American Journal of Psychology 9507–9533.

Tulving E (1985) Memory and consciousness. Canadian Psychology 26: 1–26.

Tulving, E (1993) Self knowledge of an amnesic individual is represented abstractly. In Srull TK, Wyer RS (1993) The Mental Representation of Trait and Autobiographical

Knowledge about the Self. Advances in Social Cognition 5. Hillsdale NJ: Lawrence Erlbaum 147–57.

Tyerman A, Humphrey M (1984) Changes in self concept following head injury. International Journal of Rehabilitation Research 7(1): 11–23.

Wahrborg P (1991 Assessment and Management of Emotional and Psychosocial Reactions to Brain Damage and Aphasia. Kibworth: Far Communication Disorders.

Watson JB (1998) Exploring the attitudes of adults who stutter. Journal of Communication Disorders 28: 143–164.

Wiig, E (1973) Counselling the adult aphasic for sexual readjustment. Rehabilitation Counselling Bulletin 17(2): 110–19.

Wiles A (1997) Cluttering: a case report. Unpublished student dissertation. University of Sheffield.

Wiles A, Brumfitt SM, Cowell PE (1997) A single case study of a man with cluttering difficulties. University of Sheffield, unpublished.

Williams D (1963) The problem of stuttering. In Johnson W, Darley FL, Spriestersbach DC. Diagnostic methods in speech pathology. New York. Harper and Row.

Winter DA (1992) Personal Construct Psychology in Clinical Practice. London: Routledge.

Winter D, Gourney K (1987) Constriction and construction in agoraphobia. British Journal of Medical Psychology 60: 233–44.

Wood J (1980) The language of disablement: a glossary relating to disease and its consequences. Int. Rehabil. Med. 2: 86–92.

Worden JW (1982) Grief Counselling and Therapy, 2nd edn. London: Tavistock/Routledge.

World Health Organisation (1984) Health Promotion. A Discussion Document on Concepts and Principles. Copenhagen: Regional Office for Europe.

World Health Organisation (1992) International Statistical Classification of Diseases and Related Health Problems (ICD-10). Geneva: World Health Organisation.

Worthington J (1989) The impact of adolescent development on recovery from traumatic brain injury. Rehabilitation Nursing 14(3): 118–23.

Young L, Humphrey M (1985) Cognitive methods of preparing women for hysterectomy: does a booklet help? British Journal of Clinical Psychology 24: 203–4.

Zurcher LA (1977) The Mutable Self: A Self Concept for Social Change. Beverly Hills CA: Sage.

Index